THE
ALKALINE
5 DIET

THE ALKALINE 5 DIET

Lose Weight, Heal Your Health Problems and Feel Amazing!

LAURA WILSON

HAY HOUSE

Carlsbad, California • New York City • London • Sydney
Johannesburg • Vancouver • Hong Kong • New Delhi

Dedicated to my parents,
Catherine and Keith,
and to God.

First published and distributed in the United Kingdom by:
Hay House UK Ltd, Astley House, 33 Notting Hill Gate, London W11 3JQ
Tel: +44 (0)20 3675 2450; Fax: +44 (0)20 3675 2451; www.hayhouse.co.uk

Published and distributed in the United States of America by:
Hay House Inc., PO Box 5100, Carlsbad, CA 92018-5100
Tel: (1) 760 431 7695 or (800) 654 5126
Fax: (1) 760 431 6948 or (800) 650 5115; www.hayhouse.com

Published and distributed in Australia by:
Hay House Australia Ltd, 18/36 Ralph St, Alexandria NSW 2015
Tel: (61) 2 9669 4299; Fax: (61) 2 9669 4144; www.hayhouse.com.au

Published and distributed in the Republic of South Africa by:
Hay House SA (Pty) Ltd, PO Box 990, Witkoppen 2068
info@hayhouse.co.za; www.hayhouse.co.za

Published and distributed in India by:
Hay House Publishers India, Muskaan Complex, Plot No.3, B-2,
Vasant Kunj, New Delhi 110 070
Tel: (91) 11 4176 1620; Fax: (91) 11 4176 1630; www.hayhouse.co.in

Distributed in Canada by:
Raincoast Books, 2440 Viking Way, Richmond, B.C. V6V 1N2
Tel: (1) 604 448 7100; *Fax:* (1) 604 270 7161; www.raincoast.com

Text © Laura Wilson, 2015

The information given in this book should not be treated as a substitute for
professional medical advice; always consult a medical practitioner. Any
use of information in this book is at the reader's discretion and risk. Neither
the author nor the publisher can be held responsible for any loss, claim or
damage arising out of the use, or misuse, of the suggestions made, the failure
to take medical advice or for any material on third party websites.

A catalogue record for this book is available from the British Library.

ISBN: 978-1-78180-482-7

Interior images: 51, 127, 173 © Charlie McKay; 53 © Laura Wilson

Printed and bound in Great Britain by TJ International Ltd, Padstow, Cornwall

Contents

Acknowledgements

I'd like to thank God for giving me the courage, the vision and the right words to bring this message of preventative health through a plant-based alkaline diet to the world.

Thanks to my dad, Keith, for believing in me, adopting this diet and being a great advocate of it. Thanks also to my website subscribers and clients; our work together, your feedback and your health improvements have inspired me tremendously.

I acknowledge Dr Neal Barnard, Dr John McDougall, Jason Vale, Harley and Freelee, and Anthony Robbins for their pioneering work in this area of health.

Personal thanks for their help and encouragement go to my mum, Cathy; Naso; Tom and various other family and friends. Finally, great thanks to my publisher and editors.

Foreword

For health advocates like Laura and me, there is excitement in the air. If you are reading this book, I am excited for you. Though Western countries are still burdened with obesity, diabetes, heart disease and other diet-related diseases, knowledge that a plant-based diet can combat these diseases is spreading like wildfire. The more we learn, and the more we put this knowledge into practice, the better off we will be.

When I founded the Physicians Committee in 1985, few doctors were advocating a low-fat, vegan diet for health. Today, thousands of doctors, dietitians, nurses and other healthcare professionals promote a plant-based diet. Research studies showing that fruits, vegetables, whole grains and legumes promote better health continue to be published day by day, confirming that plants are the optimal source of nutrition. In our studies at the Physicians Committee, we've seen a low-fat vegan diet reverse diabetes, bring on weight loss, lower cholesterol and blood pressure, eliminate migraines, help workplaces reduce their employee healthcare costs, and so much more. The power that a plant-based diet can have on health is simply astounding. And I am glad to see that this knowledge is spreading.

Every day, more and more people are taking meat off their grocery lists. The USDA's latest figures indicate that meat consumption is currently the lowest it has been in three decades. In the past ten years alone, Americans have dropped an average of 9kg (20lbs) of meat per year from their diets. And between 2009 and 2012, the number of people following vegan diets doubled. If we continue at this pace – and, more likely, an increased pace – our world's health will be revolutionized.

Switching to a plant-based diet helps more than our health. It also helps the Earth. Eating meat accounts for more greenhouse gases than all transportation worldwide. In fact, a recent analysis by Worldwatch Institute found that eating animals and their by-products accounts for 51% of global warming. We also lose more land space and resources by supporting the livestock industry – animals that we 'grow' to eat consume seven times more grain than the entire US population! Think how much land we could save, and how many hungry mouths we could feed, with all of that food. Not to mention, when we eat a plant-based diet, we spare the lives of animals. Eating a vegan diet saves roughly 200 animals' lives per person per year. Putting plants on your plate won't just benefit you, but also the planet and all who live here.

Of course, everyone needs a bit of help getting started. And that's okay. This is one reason that 3-week programmes like the meal plan in this book, or our 21-day Kickstart, are so effective. Three weeks gives you enough time to test-drive this new way of eating and really experience what it has to offer. In three weeks' time, your taste buds will change to appreciate, and actually prefer, fresh wholefoods. Three weeks also gives you a chance to see effects such as weight loss (if you are trying to lose weight), higher energy levels, better digestion and more. So give it a try! Use Laura's meal plan to guide you, and see what you think. I have a good feeling you'll enjoy it.

Dr Neal D. Barnard

Founder and president of the Physicians Committee for Responsible Medicine (PCRM), and author of *Power Foods for the Brain*.

Introduction

Welcome to Abundance, Balance and Harmony

I am so excited that you've picked up this book because I have seen how this diet can change lives for the better. So if, like many people, you yearn to look and feel your best, or are struggling with a health challenge and have lost faith in the possibility of ever healing yourself, then you've arrived at the right place, because the road to feeling fantastic starts here. Thousands of other people are already enjoying the results of following the Alkaline 5 Diet (A5D), and my hope is that you too will find that following the diet for just three weeks will be transformative to your health, your eating and your relationship with food.

So get ready for a truly great experience.

The principles of the Alkaline 5 Diet (A5D) are simple: abundance, balance and working in harmony with your body's nutritional needs. However, there is more to a healthy lifestyle than just food, so the A5D takes care of your emotional wellbeing, fitness and rest needs too. Taking care of both your physical *and* your emotional needs means that at the end of the 21 days, you'll not only be in the best shape ever, but also be radiant and glowing with energy, calm and confidence – so much so that other people will comment on how great you look.

The Alkaline 5 Diet is grounded in solid science and has a simplicity to it that makes it unique in the landscape of all-too-common faddy, restrictive, pseudo-healthy diets. This is because A5D is the diet that humans were designed to eat and, for that reason, it's satisfying on many different levels.

In Part III, you'll get a clear 21-day meal plan and using the diet for just three weeks will return your body to a more natural, healthier state. From that point, it's likely that you'll be able to delight in a simpler, yet deliciously tasty, way of eating; one you may not have experienced before and that's free of cravings and hunger. Using the diet may also change how you think and feel about food, and many people find that they adopt some of, if not all, the meal types and ways of eating long into the future.

> *I had no idea that my decision to follow the Alkaline 5 Diet would change my life so much for the better. All my health issues went away within a few months – and I had a fair few – I also became so much happier. Now I look at the world from a more positive perspective and the 55lb weight loss is really just an added bonus!* – GRETA

I have been using the Alkaline 5 Diet for many years and it has allowed me a level of health and vibrancy beyond that of the vast majority of people. Here are the benefits of following A5D for 21 days:

♦ Fat loss, usually 3.5–9kgs (8–20lbs).

♦ Greater vibrancy and sustained energy throughout the day.

- Positive mindset and a general sense of calm, happiness and wellbeing.

- An improvement in any health issues you may have.

    I have lost 9lbs in the past 21 days and feel amazing, thank you, Laura! – Tracy

When you follow the A5D over the longer term – for three months or more – you may also experience the following:

- Looking and feeling years younger than your actual age.

- Active signs of age-reversal: toned and blemish-free skin, eyes that look whiter and brighter, and shiny healthy-looking hair.

- Excellent fitness and recovery.

- Balanced hormones.

- Reversal of minor and even major health issues and diseases.

- Improved body tone and muscle definition.

Today's reality

We live in a world like never before. The Internet has changed how many of us live, shop, socialize and access information – forever. The new paradigm of the world is infinite instant choice, and this has its good and bad attributes.

On the one hand, we can type anything we want into an online browser and find thousands of pages of information to answer our query, or find what to buy – and the cheapest place to buy it – and have it delivered the next day, which is pretty incredible when you think about it.

On the other hand, however, we can also become information overloaded – bombarded with messages, alerts, pings, emails, updates, phone calls, videos and advertisements. Unchecked, it's easy to spend all day long just reacting to the incoming information around us, rather than actually making considered choices and being truly productive. Everything is fast – fast information, faster travel, fast food, fast eating – and this brings with it some negative consequences.

With so many choices and options, instant availability and information overload, we can get pulled all over the place and lose track of the most important things. Ironically, too much choice can be like having no choice at all – we can become confused, caught up and just end up going with what's easiest and grabbing our attention right now, rather than right for us. What's more, fast information and living often leads to having a slow body – sat in front of computers, devices and TV screens instead of being out walking and exercising.

The result? Western societies are now facing huge problems: many people are now overweight or obese; preventable disease is rife – cancer, heart disease and diabetes are major causes of death; lifestyles are characterized by stress, long working hours and trying to keep afloat in the economic crisis, which all adds up to just existing rather than living.

According to statistics published by the World Health Organization, more than 1.4 billion adults, aged 20 and older, were overweight at the time of the study (this could be even more now). Of these, more than 200 million men and nearly 300 million women were obese.[1]

We are also taught to devolve our power. Feeling ill or stressed? Take a pill. Got no cash? Borrow to the hilt (look what happened with that). The media and governments tell us that everything is bad and that this is normal.

I am here to tell you that *this is not normal!*

It is absolutely within your power to have an abundant, happy and healthy lifestyle. As Ralph Waldo Emerson said, 'The first wealth is health', and so the first step in reclaiming your power is about taking care of your health by nurturing your body and making smart food and lifestyle choices. This book is about just that.

The new model and opportunity

One definite major benefit of the Internet, and having unparalleled access to information, is that we can find out about our health and wellbeing, and make more informed choices. Thanks to online information, many more people are now aware of alternative medicine and health options, which are not presented in the mainstream media. Obviously we have to choose our sources of information wisely and do due diligence, but there is a shift towards self-diagnosis and self-doctoring, as we have an elevated awareness of our health needs and the science of wellbeing.

It's also true that many people have lost faith in the advice given by traditional authority figures, such as the government and medical professionals – particularly since we are seeing economic and health crises all around the globe. Intuitively, we are looking for alternative, improved, trustworthy guidance and leadership.

The net result: we are more intelligent and empowered. We are no longer prepared to settle for second-rate and are demanding higher standards of health. Since you are reading this book, I know that you are also one of these people. I know this to be true because I get emails every day from many of my 15,000-plus website subscribers seeking ways to improve their health and overall quality of life.

The new model of reality is one of consumer power. After all, if we are unsatisfied with something, anything, at the click of a button we can send our views to the world via social media. Furthermore, we can seek advice to challenges from a collective online community of friends and gurus.

Knowledge about alkaline diets is part of this new model and awareness. In the 15 or so years since I set up my first alkaline diet website and wrote my first books and articles on the subject, I have connected with many other people who are also informed about the powerful benefits of an alkaline diet and the benefits of drinking wheatgrass juice or following a raw diet, for example. So the new opportunity is this: we have the information and support to help us lead our best lives – healthy and vibrant – at our fingertips.

Anthony Robbins, a hugely respected US life coach and author of many bestselling books on personal power, emphatically advocates 'getting the edge' in life and achieving 'supreme health power' by eating a predominantly raw and plant-based diet, while other respected authors and doctors, such as John McDougall and Neal Barnard, advocate a holistic approach to health; and many expert nutritionists, such as Jason Vale, advocate juices and smoothies for great health.

It has been said that with great power comes great responsibility and this is no exception. We must take the initiative to nurture our own and our loved ones' health. Reading this book will help you to increase your power. In return it is important to take responsibility for your health and commit to living your best life, starting today, no matter how old, young, ill, bored, happy, unhappy, apathetic you may have been prior to this point. The amusing paradox is that to commit and take responsibility leads to greater freedom and isn't that what we all desire?

So armed with the knowledge you gain from this book, seize the new opportunity – grab on to the possibility of your supreme health and life with both hands and go get it!

Is 'supreme health' really possible for me?

If you're asking this question, then I totally get how you're feeling because I used to ask it too. I used to be unfit, a smoker, a bit overweight, totally lethargic, regularly get illnesses and felt pretty awful most of the time… and I was in my early twenties. In fact I felt like this from 16 to 21 years of age.

I remember having friends at school that were very sporty – one who was an Olympic swimmer and others that were brilliant at basketball, hockey or athletics. I was pretty good at badminton, but when it came to the team sports I was usually picked last. Stupidly, I started smoking, eating badly and losing fitness and vitality; and this trend continued when I went to university. I am embarrassed to say that I became known as 'The Pot Noodle Kid' – not a great reputation to have and a far cry from where I am today.

Now I am very fit and healthy. I have energy to do the things I really love: run long-distance, complete marathons and ultra-marathon endurance races with very respectable times; dance salsa for hours on end; and sing two-hour live concerts as a soprano member of a classical philharmonic choir. On top of that, I look youthful and feel vibrant and happy.

So if you are asking 'Is this really possible for me?' Then, yes, absolutely! You can do this. You can have the health, vitality, joy, self-esteem and happiness that you deserve and it won't take long to start seeing great results either.

The secret

The simple secret to great health lies in keeping your body alkaline. Alkaline foods, such as raw leafy greens, enhance your body and brain chemistry. Enhanced body and brain chemistry fosters positive emotions such as happiness, enthusiasm and hope, which are, in turn, alkaline.

When you start detoxifying your body of acidity, it is difficult to be unhappy and unhealthy, and the good news is that you can choose to do something alkaline for your body next week, tomorrow or right now. For example, deep breathing clean fresh air is alkaline. Furthermore, your body, being the amazingly intelligent thing it is, will respond positively and almost immediately to the new and enhanced choices you make and fuel that you provide it.

If you are sceptical, imagine the following Friday-night scenario:

One person chooses to drink a few glasses of wine and then goes out to a club with work colleagues, commiserates with them about the unfairness of the management team, has a few more drinks, eats a greasy Indian curry, sees a drunken fight on the way home before going to bed at 3 a.m. and getting five hours' sleep.

The other person goes for a walk in the local park after work and takes some time to reflect on the past week and enjoy nature; goes home and rings a friend whom they haven't seen for a while, and laughs about old times; reads a chapter of an uplifting book whilst drinking a cup of herbal tea; and has an early night, sleeping for eight hours.

On Saturday morning, who is likely to feel better and healthier? The first person is likely to feel dehydrated, tired, hungover; and with a fuzzy mindset at best and a depressed mindset at worst. The second person is likely to feel refreshed, healthy, calm and ready to take on the new day with enthusiasm.

It's self-evident that the different decisions we take today have vastly different consequences for how tomorrow pans out. So imagine making better-quality decisions on a day-to-day basis. They don't have to be huge. Just making small shifts here and there will make a massive difference over the long term. In the same way that changing a ship's direction by one compass point makes hundreds of miles' difference in destination over its entire course.

In this book, we'll be exploring how to achieve great health in an unhealthy world, based on the 'Seven-Point Framework for Optimum Health and Healing', which I developed in 2008 and have since seen help thousands of people to create healthier lifestyles.

I am going to show you some simple, quick and practical ways to become more alkaline – and therefore more vibrant and healthy – so that you can do it any time for an instant boost. You will discover:

♦   Morning rituals to give you an instant kick.

♦   Simple ways to eliminate stress and keep your mind on what you want in life, rather than what you don't want.

♦   How to identify alkaline foods from acidic foods; and the truth behind why a lot of 'alkaline food lists' differ.

♦ Powerhouse foods, which are great for vitality, but also improve concentration, fertility, anti-ageing, detoxification, libido, spiritual connectedness, healing, sleep and much more.

♦ The 21-day Alkaline 5 Diet meal plan, which will show you how to eat for supreme health, healing, beauty and energy.

♦ Useful resources to help you succeed on this diet and take it to the next level once you've finished the book.

So keep reading.

I started eating predominately alkaline foods to help with my stomach condition. I am having good results so far, and am hoping to do without meds soon. I have been largely veggie for years now so don't think there'll be too much of a transition problem… it's really just about ingraining it now. I am feeling great at the moment and it's pretty easy. – CATHY

Chapter 1

The Good and Bad News about Diet and Health

'Diet' and 'health' are rather ambiguous terms because they can mean so many different things to people, and throw up lots of different emotions, feelings and connections to personal experiences and beliefs. In fact, it's hard to think of any words that are as powerfully emotive, except for a handful of others such as 'love', 'family', 'war', 'religion' and 'fear'.

Many people think of diet as meaning deprivation, hunger and blandness, and often prefix it with the term 'yo-yo' to denote the common pattern of starving and losing weight, followed by bingeing and weight gain. However, when I use the term 'diet' in this book, as in the Alkaline 5 Diet, it is intended in a much more neutral way; it means the foods we eat to sustain ourselves.

So, before starting out, it is important to let go of any emotional ties or past-held beliefs or faddy notions (or those supported by the food industry and media for that matter) that you have about the word 'diet'. Instead, think about it as a way of describing functional body fuel. No more, no less.

The word 'health' is similarly ambiguous and emotionally loaded. Health, in my view, is more than the absence of disease. I define it is as the Five Elements of Great Health, which are as follows:

1. Absence of both physical and mental disease and ailments.

2. A strong, energized and fit body that is neither underweight nor overweight.

3. An open mind that experiences a full range of emotions, in which positivity and a sense of purpose in life dominate.

4. An overriding sense of security in the ability to handle the challenges that life throws at us, and therefore an absence of negative stress.

5. An enthusiasm for, and sense of connection to, the world, people and our spiritual self.

Great health is elusive for most people and, for many others, achieving all of the five elements seems near impossible. Let's face it, the current state of human health, as a whole species, is in turmoil. We won't dwell on this too much, but just consider for a moment the following facts.

♦ On our planet, millions of people (in fact, 80 per cent of the world's population) right now are starving, undernourished and without proper sanitation, water and everyday amenities; they are simply fighting to stay alive.

♦ There are also millions of people (in the other 20 per cent), who are overfed, overweight or obese, ill, unfit, have body image issues and are also undernourished.

◆ In our current technological and industrial age, we have access to all the information, guidance, advice, support, correct nutrition and food we could ever possibly need and desire – for the whole human race – yet more and more people are becoming diseased, obese and even dying prematurely of cancer, heart disease, diabetes, stroke and many other preventable diseases, brought on largely by detrimental lifestyle choices.

How can this be? What is going on here?

The 'health' agenda

Giant corporations (soda producers, fast food restaurants, processed-food manufacturers, pharmaceutical companies) fund health research and the setting of erroneous government recommended daily allowances for fat, protein and carbohydrates.[1,2] Take the food industry regulatory bodies and world's governments for example, who are lobbied and funded by the meat and dairy industries.[3] What does this tell you?

You're an intelligent person; I'll let you draw your own conclusions.

Whilst it's noble and trusting to believe that we can put our faith in 'the system', when it comes to our diet and health, it would be deadly to do so; and the disease facts and figures reflect this. Currently, one in three people get cancer, a disease that is wholly preventable. It has been shown that genetic factors play a very small part in many diseases – around 3 per cent,[4] the research shows. Ultimately your health is *your* responsibility.

The game has changed

These days many foods are, or contain ingredients that are, genetically modified (GMO) – soya (soy), grains, animal products and virtually any and all processed packaged foods and sauces. The problem is that GMO foods have not been around long enough for us to know the full ramifications of eating such unnatural foods. However, we do know that they have been shown to have adverse effects on health in many different ways, from sparking gluten intolerances, to breast cancer and birth defects.[5–9] We are living in a world in which unscrupulous food giants are seriously compromising our health. Therefore the easiest way to ensure your good health and avoid GMOs is to adopt a plant-based diet and buy organic produce whenever possible.

My aim in this book is to help you decipher the 'health messages' that we're bombarded with daily via the media and Internet, so that you never have to worry and wonder again about what is the best diet for you. I have spent 15 years reading, researching, experimenting and getting feedback from my website subscribers about all aspects of diet and fitness.

Of course, you don't have to take my word for it and I highly recommend that you also do your own research. Watch the documentaries I recommend, then watch the ones saying the opposite – the Paleo diet and the Atkins diet – and look at what these people are promoting; look at their health, physique, vibrancy and fitness (or lack of these things) and make your own conclusions, based on your instinct.

I believe that the Alkaline 5 Diet is the perfect diet for humans and all of the REAL evidence backs it up. My request, however, is that you simply try it for 21 days and then judge for yourself, based on your own experience.

Having studied nutrition since 1999 and worked in medical-research management (as well as having applied good health principles to my life and had the privilege to help others around the world do the same), I have found beliefs and practices around health are *divergent*. The mainstream view advocated dubiously as fact by the mass media, and the health, food and pharmaceutical industries, and the alternative or enlightened view advocated by natural health practitioners, followers and industries whose main priority and goal is great health – not related to or dependent on funding, sales targets, politics and sensationalism.

Mainstream beliefs about health

♦ Good or bad health is determined largely by our genes and to a lesser extent by our diet and lifestyle. Diseases such as cancer are unfortunate and strike randomly and without warning, often without an obvious cause.

♦ Medical researchers are working very hard to discover new and ground-breaking techniques and medicines to fight cancer, which will help us all and cure diseases.

♦ The most effective and logical way of addressing disease is with drugs, most of which manage disease but do not cure it.

♦ A good diet includes five fruits and vegetables per day (can be cooked, tinned, frozen or fresh), balanced with whole grains, legumes and pulses and smaller quantities of animal proteins and dairy products. Low-fat and 'healthy-fat' foods are good and we should avoid too much sugar and simple carbohydrates.

♦ Moderate exercise is advised – three to five 30-minute sessions of light exercise (walking or gentle cycling, swimming etc.) per week is ideal.

♦ We are all under a lot of stress, but this is just the way it is. The economic crisis has brought with it uncertainty, and that means we are all in the same boat and just need to get on with it as best we can – that's life.

Enlightened beliefs about health

♦ Good or bad health is determined largely by the foods we eat and the lifestyle choices we make. This plays a vastly more important role in determining health than genetics. Therefore the fate of our health lies firmly with us. We reap what we sow; it's an inescapable and universal law.

♦ All disease, including cancer, is the body's way of dealing with *over-acidity* in the cells. It is not random, but a natural reaction to acidosis and has a distinct cause and effect. There is no 'cure for cancer'. This is a myth that the pharmaceutical industry promotes in order to keep selling drugs. The cure for cancer and all other diseases is to restore the body's pH balance. As Dr Otto Warburg (Nobel Prize winner in 1931) discovered, disease cannot thrive in an alkaline environment. This is the 'cure'.[10]

♦ The best and most logical way of addressing a disease or illness is *not* with drugs or surgical procedures – these often only mask the symptoms and do not address the root cause. Often these medical interventions can worsen the problems, as drugs produce side effects and so greater acidity in the body. The best and most logical way to address a disease or illness is to provide our infinitely intelligent body with the correct nutrition, oxygen, hydration, rest, exercise and positive emotions it requires to *heal itself*.

♦ Good diet is predominantly an alkaline one, which should include 8 to 20 organic fruits and vegetables per day (preferably raw, not cooked, tinned or frozen), balanced with energy-giving starches, such as rice, and other whole grains, potatoes, pasta, quinoa and root vegetables. We should avoid refined oils, animal and dairy products, as well as packaged and processed foods.

♦ Exercise is advised – three to five sessions per week of cardiovascular and short, anaerobic, high-intensity exercise is recommended for a great level of fitness.

♦ We should live relatively stress-free lives. There is no need to be stressed out; it's not what life is about and stress is a choice because we can choose our attitude to events and circumstances. We have control over our lives, including our finances, happiness and health. If something is not working, it is our responsibility, and within our power, to change it.

What is an alkaline diet?

The alkaline diet is based around the pH scale, which was developed in 1909 by Danish chemist Søren Peder Lauritz Sørensen.[11] The term pH stands for 'potential of hydrogen' because it measures the number of hydrogen ions in a standard volume of liquid. Therefore the acidity or alkalinity of a substance is determined by the concentration of hydrogen ions (positively charged hydrogen molecules). An acid is a substance that is saturated with hydrogen ions, while an alkali (or base) is a substance that is capable of absorbing many hydrogen ions.

An alkaline diet is a healthy-eating lifestyle based on eating foods that metabolize (burn) to leave an alkaline residue (ash) of minerals such as calcium, iron, zinc, magnesium and copper. Foods are therefore classified as alkaline, acidic or neutral according to the pH of the solution created with their ash in water. Acidity and alkalinity are measured using the pH (potential of hydrogen) scale, which spans from zero to 14, with zero being the most acidic, 14 the most alkaline and 7 as neutral.

Our body's tissues each have an optimal pH range that they need to maintain for good functioning: muscle tissue needs a pH of 6.1, the liver 6.9, the stomach 1.2–3.0, the urine 4.5–8.0, the saliva 6.35–6.85, and the blood 7.35–7.45, etc. When we deviate from these optimal ranges, problems arise and the body takes emergency measures to restore it to the optimal set point (called homeostasis). Your body has a 'buffer' system that it uses to keep your blood within a tight range of this pH, a deviation from which can be fatal.

Blood is the largest tissue in the body and it is also the most important in sustaining life. It transports oxygen (via red blood corpuscles), nutrients and water to our cells. It also eliminates acidic waste that builds up during cellular processes. The blood is often called our 'river of life', and less important functions in the body will be compromised in order to restore correct blood pH. In chronic acidosis, alkaline minerals are drawn from the body to maintain life-sustaining blood pH.[12,13]

The three predominant alkaline minerals are sodium, calcium and potassium, which are recycled by the kidneys back into the blood and lymph by binding them to carbon dioxide. For example, the body will borrow (leech) calcium and other alkaline minerals from our bones, muscles and vital organs to neutralize blood acidity. This literally saves our life in the short term, but at the expense of compromised bone health (leading possibly to osteoporosis) over the longer term.[14]

The alkaline pH balance diet is concerned with working in harmony with your body's requirements for healthy functioning – namely, keeping your blood pH at its optimal, slightly alkaline range of 7.35–7.45, without any stress on other functions and mineral reserves. This is achieved predominantly by eating foods that create an alkaline ash when metabolized by the body – fruit and vegetables – and limiting foods which create an acidic ash – such as animal products, dairy, refined oils and processed foods.

❧ Alkaline-delicious tip ❧

The alkalinity of your body has nothing to do with your stomach acid or even the pH of foods in their physical form. For example, lemons are alkaline-forming but acidic in their physical form.

How does an alkaline diet work?

You can determine you body's pH by testing your saliva and urine pH using litmus paper or pH strips that can be bought online or from health food stores very inexpensively. Check your saliva and urine pH level first thing in the morning and just before going to sleep at night. Since we do not eat through the night, the morning saliva and urine pH indicate the acidity of the body. Evening saliva and urine pH show how our diet and lifestyle influences our metabolism and how well our buffer systems are tolerating the changing pH. The saliva and urine pH offer a window through which you can see the overall pH balance in your body.

This is useful because even if you usually feel fine, if your diet consists mostly of meat, packaged foods, caffeine, dairy, refined fats and sugars, or you are constantly under stress, do not exercise enough, smoke, or drink alcohol, your saliva and urine pH will probably register as low as 5.0–6.0 on the pH scale and this is an early warning indicator that you need to make some immediate changes to alkalize your body.

Over-acidity can go undetected for years, but causes severe damage and will eventually manifest into a significant health problem. Like acid eating into marble, acidosis erodes and eats into cell wall membranes of the heart, arteries and veins. Acidosis is the first step towards having a weakened immune function, premature ageing and chronic disease.

The easiest way to maintain correct blood pH is by following an alkaline diet[15] and lifestyle that works in harmony with your body's needs. Drinking water also helps to maintain alkalinity in the blood, lymph, intracellular and extracellular fluids, by diluting excess acidity.

So in essence, the simple and obvious reasoning behind the alkaline diet is one of being an ally, a friend and a champion to your body's natural requirements and healthy state of being, so it can get on with carrying out its multitude of functions and processes, unobstructed and using the correct fuel.

Think of it like this – providing alkaline foods to your body is like fuelling your racing car with high-octane petrol (gas) and running it on a racetrack with no obstacles. You wouldn't fuel your racing car with diesel and put breeze blocks on the road, so why on earth would you do this to your body?

Awareness of the alkaline diet

The alkaline diet is really nothing new. After all, everyone can appreciate the sense in eating more vegetables and less junk food. The term 'alkaline diet' has been around since the early 1920s, when New York physician William Howard Hay introduced the world to the Hay Diet (although in a somewhat erroneous way, many would argue) and its results of helping people to heal and find great health are well documented.

From 1909, Ann Wigmore and the Hippocrates Health Institute published *Why Suffer? Be Your Own Doctor*, *The Healing Power Within* and *Recipes for Longer Life*[16], which gives numerous and practical examples of how wheatgrass – a hugely beneficial alkaline superfood, which you'll learn more about shortly – and other organic raw greens can be, and have been, used to reverse terminal illness. Ann Wigmore documented thousands of positive case studies of patients at the Institute and in her books.

Despite the best efforts of mainstream society to label raw-food and vegan diets as 'hippyish' and 'extreme', these approaches to diet and health have gained a lot in popularity since the sixties and the alkaline diet has become similarly more popular, especially in the last 10 years.

Although the basic concept behind the alkaline diet has been around for almost a century, it broke into the mainstream with the publication of Dr Robert O Young's *The pH Miracle* in 2003. This ground-breaking book talks about the 'new biology of health' and addresses the benefits of correct food combining. Transitioning into an alkaline diet of 80:20 alkaline-acidic foods can overcome an array of common health issues and diseases, which as we know, afflict a huge number of people living in the developed world.

Since then the alkaline diet has been gaining momentum and many other publications have been written advocating its health benefits; it has also received a lot of airtime at events such as Anthony Robbins' *Unleash the Power Within* seminars.

It is my view that in a few years' time, the alkaline diet will be mainstream and most people will have heard of it and will strive to alkalize more. It will go from being an 'underground' diet to commonplace.

Is the alkaline diet the same as a vegan diet?

An alkaline diet is concerned with eating 80 per cent or more of your calories from alkaline foods, such as fruits, vegetables, grains and pulses, to work in harmony with your body's optimal pH balance. A vegan diet is concerned with eating only plant-based foods and eliminating all meat and dairy products, usually for ethical reasons.

Both are great diets, yet it is still possible to be unhealthy on both. No doubt everyone knows a vegetarian or vegan who drinks soda drinks and alcohol, and eats microwave meals, and there are advocates of the alkaline diet who regularly eat acidic meat, cheese or fish. Therefore, the very best diet is one that combines the good principles of both the alkaline diet and a vegan diet.

Alkaline *and* vegan means eliminating animal products (meat, fish, dairy, eggs and honey) altogether, as well as other highly acidic foods, and eating a diet high in fresh, ripe fruits and vegetables. This is really the holy grail of achieving great health, a lean body and greater energy, preventing and reversing disease and looking and feeling your best.

Thus the Alkaline 5 Diet is both alkaline and vegan. In the 21-day diet we'll be aiming for a 70:30 ratio of alkaline–acidic foods/drinks (or 80:20 if you want to be stricter), as this is the optimum balance.[17–19]

A5D is also about eliminating, or at least limiting, acidifying toxins such as parabens found in beauty products and plastics, the harmful 'radiolytic' toxins produced by microwave ovens, not smoking, not drinking alcohol (or drinking very sparingly) and avoiding negative and acidifying emotions such as stress.

These are health fundamentals, not the latest 'diet of the day', which is why the alkaline diet is *the best diet* for humans and is totally sustainable over the long term. In fact, the longer you stick with an alkaline diet the more positive results you'll reap.

The Paleo Diet™, the ketone diet, the Dukan Diet, and various other high-protein or high-fat diets, will NOT produce health. They may cause you to lose weight in the short term, but this is at the expense of the health of your organs – in particular your kidneys,[20–21] as my friend Kathy's story demonstrates.

I met Kathy when I was at the Thailand Fruit Festival recently. She had been following an alkaline vegan diet (eating only fruits and vegetables) and having great health results. She told me the story of how, in her younger years, she was into bodybuilding and followed a high-protein and meat-based diet. She was lean and fit and outwardly looked pretty great. All the while and unbeknown to her, however, this diet was wreaking havoc on her kidneys. She began to experience some major health problems and found out that her kidney function had reduced to just 30 per cent, and that she needed immediate kidney dialysis. She eventually had to have an operation to give her an extra kidney (she now has three) and a whole host of steroids and other drugs (14 per day) to manage all of this.

Since following an alkaline plant-based diet, her kidney function has returned to 90 per cent and she's off the majority of her drugs. Her doctors say it's 'inexplicable' and she's 'lucky'. Kathy knows it's down to her diet and lifestyle and she says she feels fantastic.

The statements I've made here may sound very bold and go against what you might otherwise have been taught or conditioned to believe, and I encourage you not simply to take my word for it. Look at the numerous credible studies and work (i.e. not funded by pharmaceutical or food industries) by pioneering researchers such as Dr Neal Barnard, Dr T. Colin Campbell and Dr Caldwell Esselstyn.

Clinical researcher and author Dr Neal Barnard is one of America's leading advocates for health nutrition and is founder of the Physicians Committee for Responsible Medicine (PCRM). He has been published in several peer-reviewed medical and scientific journals and written many ground-breaking books, such as *The Get Healthy, Go Vegan Cookbook: 125 Easy and Delicious Recipes to Jump-Start Weight Loss and Help You Feel Great; Dr Neal Barnard's Program for Reversing Diabetes;* and *Breaking the Food Seduction.*

Dr T. Colin Campbell wrote the book *The China Study*, which is based on the China-Cornell-Oxford Project, a 20-year scientific study into health. It examined the relationship between eating meat and dairy products and chronic illnesses such as diabetes, heart disease and cancers of the breast, prostate and bowel. It showed that people who eat a wholefood, vegan diet – avoiding all animal products and reducing their intake of processed foods and refined carbohydrates – will escape, reduce or reverse the development of numerous diseases.

Dr Caldwell Esselstyn has conducted extensive research into a plant-based diet for reversing heart disease and has published more than 150 scientific papers. His book *Prevent and Reverse Heart Disease* is based on his 20-year study, proving changes in diet and nutrition can actually cure heart disease.

I would advise that you read at least one of the books by these world-leading nutrition researchers and practitioners.

The common theme of these doctors' research is that they advocate cutting *all* animal products from our diet and keeping it low fat. By its nature, a diet devoid of animal products automatically cuts out a large percentage of saturated fat. Therefore, the best diet is one that is alkaline and also vegan.

Benefits of a low-fat vegan diet

The alkaline plant-based diet has many medically and scientifically documented benefits to health and wellbeing. Each week I receive lots of emails from my website subscribers telling me that since changing to a low-fat vegan diet, their skin problems have cleared up, they've lost excess weight, some have come off hay fever or asthma medication, reversed diabetes and even seen more astonishing improvements in serious diseases, such as cancer and heart disease.

Unfortunately there are people in positions of power whose interests are not served by this kind of information, i.e. simple solutions to common health problems. However, there is an extensive body of data, proof, studies and evidence to show that a low-fat vegan diet is best. You just won't find it on TV or in the press very often. Let's hope that changes.

One of the most amazing benefits of following this lifestyle is how quickly you begin to see health improvements and generally feel better. Because it's the diet us humans are supposed to be on, once we start alkalizing, our bodies go straight to work 'cleaning house' and replenishing our cells.

It is almost certain that when you switch to the Alkaline 5 Diet from acidic foods, after a few days of detox symptoms – such as tiredness, headaches, mild dizziness – you'll start to see some good shifts in energy, weight, skin condition, mood, concentration and more.

Many people are concerned about getting enough protein on a vegan diet, but they needn't be – plants are actually a superior source.[22]

Proteins are made from chains of 20 different amino acids that connect together in varying sequences. Plants (and microorganisms) can synthesize all of the individual amino acids that are used to build proteins, but animals cannot. There are eight amino acids that people cannot make, and thus these must be obtained from our diets – they are referred to as 'essential'.

We actually require very little protein – 5 per cent of our calories from protein is recommended by the World Health Organization (WHO). This quantity of protein is impossible to avoid when you eat a fruit-and-vegetable-based diet. Certainly A5D covers more than enough of your protein needs – you'll be getting around 10 per cent of your daily calories from protein, which is optimum.

Restrictive and boring? Think again

Eating an alkaline vegan diet is actually very liberating. Think of it like driving a car. If you weren't aware of the reasoning and sense behind the concept of having to take a driving test, learn the rules of the road and follow road markings and signs, you might think that it all sounds very boring and restrictive. You might be inclined to think, 'But I just want to drive. I want to be free to do what I want, I don't want to learn rules and pass tests.'

However, if there were no clear markings on the roads and no rules for drivers, how fast would you be able to drive? How easy would it be to get to your desired destination? How much faith could you have in other drivers? How safe would you be?

The fact that there are clear *parameters* in place makes it easier for us to drive fast and be safe with ease and peace of mind. This gives us freedom, rather than taking it away.

It's the same with A5D. There are clear parameters in place so that you can move through life with great health, high energy, a lean body and a positive state of mind. This is a *high-performance* diet. If you want to get the best out of your life and have the *option* to drive in the fast lane at any given opportunity or time you wish, then this is the diet to follow.

Possible health improvements

Here are some of the health improvements that a plant-based diet can give:

♦ Prevention and reversal of disease – helping to avoid many widespread and preventable diseases such as colds and yeast infections, as well as the big three killers – heart disease, diabetes and cancer.

♦ Improved immune function.

♦ Weight loss – as your body releases excess acid stored in fat and metabolizes your food more efficiently.

♦ Slower and reversed signs of ageing as the life of your body's cells is prolonged.

♦ More energy than ever and no afternoon sluggishness.

♦ Great skin, as you no longer need to release acidic toxins through it.

♦ Better sleep.

♦ Aids a healthy libido and erectile function.

♦ Aids the body's natural healing mechanisms.

♦ Improvement in allergies.

♦ Healthier teeth and gums.

♦ More energy and vibrancy.

♦ Better mental health – feeling more positive, resilient and happier in general.

♦ Moving towards excellent health and a higher quality of life.

There's more to health than the absence of disease. This lifestyle will make you feel alive and vital – improving concentration, mental and physical stamina and overall self-esteem.

> I've only been on this diet for one week and the results are incredible. I've suffered with chronic fatigue for years, but one week on this diet and it has completely vanished. I'm only getting five to six hours sleep per night, but I am never tired. I've suffered with terrible heartburn and indigestion for years and that has vanished too. The main reason I started this diet was because I was getting pains in my

heart. Those pains have gone and I haven't experienced them once on this diet. I truly feel fantastic. I'm eating lots of fresh raw vegetables and drinking green smoothies. The Alkaline 5 Diet definitely works. – Nɪᴄᴏʟᴀ

Chapter 2

The Principles of the
Alkaline 5 Diet

A5D is not a short-term fad diet; it is designed to work over the long term and then you will reap the full benefits. By all means try it for just 21 days to start with, but if and when you are ready to make this diet your way of life, this book will help you succeed.

In a nutshell, the Alkaline 5 Diet means eating a high-fibre, high-carbohydrate, low-fat vegan (animal product-free) diet made up of lots of alkaline-forming foods such as an array of vegetables and leafy greens, fruits, potatoes and root vegetables, rice and other cooked carbohydrates. You must also drink adequate pure water – at least 2.5 litres (4½ pints) per day.

Since you bought this book, you are entitled to get a free copy of my full-colour Alkaline 5 Diet handy info-graphic that you can print and put on your wall or have on your desktop as an easy referral guide to help you succeed with A5D. You also get a free video guide that I've recorded for you. Simply go to www.Alkaline5Diet.com and use the password laurawilson.

If you'd like personal coaching to help you succeed with the Alkaline 5 Diet, through the 21 days and beyond, then do check out my website in the Resources section (see page 231). I hold regular online events and give one-to-one personal coaching that will really help support you, accelerate your results and hold you accountable.

Developing A5D

You might be wondering how I came to discover the benefits of an alkaline diet lifestyle and develop A5D. The short version is that it arose from a combination of personal struggle, using myself as a 'guinea pig', observation, reading and studying, finding what works and what doesn't through tweaking and testing new things, working as a medical research manager in the UK's health service, training as an endurance athlete, qualifying as an Advanced Gym Instructor and Registered Nutritionist, interviewing other health experts and researching relentlessly for the past 15 years – all mixed with a big dose of passion for success, excellence and desire to help other people overcome their own personal health struggles.

I have tested every diet under the sun on myself and tracked my fitness and athletic performance as an ultra-marathon runner, triathlete and dancer. I have tripped up with my diet more times than I can remember, but in doing so I have also found and honed what works consistently for great health and sustained energy.

I have interviewed many doctors and experts and helped and received feedback from my tens of thousands of website subscribers all around the world, as well as many friends and family members. Research, action, curiosity and passion led me to commit to my own lifelong pursuit of excellent fitness and health, setting up my website to help others and eventually writing two books (so far) on the alkaline diet and natural health. I also hold a large health seminar called the Natural Health and Vitality Conference, where I bring leading world experts together to present their views and experience on the path to excellent health.

This book is a culmination of everything I have learned and observed since 1995 on the subject of great health, from a wide variety of perspectives and sources. So it is worth noting that the benefits of an alkaline diet are not merely my opinion. I am simply a messenger – hopefully making these universal health laws more accessible to you and dispelling some of the myths that mass media puts in front of us about health and disease.

The reality is, having worked in both camps – mainstream medical research and natural health and nutrition – I would have to be a complete fool to miss the truth of what an optimum human diet looks like. Therefore I designed the Alkaline 5 Diet with the following criteria in mind:

♦ Systematic – easy to learn, implement and repeat to achieve consistently good results.

♦ Sustainable over the long term – you could do this diet for the next 20 years.

♦ Nutritionally complete – providing all the body's macro and micronutrient needs.

♦ Accessible and feasible in the society we live in and for whole families to adopt.

- ◆ Having an option for 100 per cent raw vegan, for people wanting the 'gold standard' fruitarian-style diet.

- ◆ Supporting both top athletic and strength performance.

- ◆ Supporting bodily regeneration and healing without the use of medical interventions.

- ◆ Convenient and with easy, quick food preparation.

- ◆ High on the scale of taste and eating satisfaction, with no calorie restriction.

The key to the success of A5D is in its simplicity. I have been following The Alkaline 5 Diet for years and love it! I am sure that within a week of doing it yourself and getting to know how it works in practice, you will love it too.

The bad news: courage, confusion and complexity

In the previous chapter, I stated that beliefs and practices around health are 'diverging'. The mainstream medicine-based health system is at one end of the spectrum and the 'enlightened', alternative, balanced nutrition-based approach is at the other.

So really, to a large extent, we have to pick a side and set of beliefs. That's not to say that the two are mutually exclusive – there is definitely a valid role to play for medicine and our traditional health services (most obviously in accident and emergency, but also to complement good nutrition in certain circumstances).

For anyone who's taken the time intelligently to find out and read about health (other than material presented by mainstream TV and media) and is also willing to accept responsibility for their own health (and not relinquish it to someone else to 'sort out' when things go wrong), it really is hard to come to any conclusion other than the enlightened nutrition-based approach to health as being the one to believe in and strive to live by.

This decision in itself is a courageous one. If you decide that your health is in your own hands and adjust your nutritional habits accordingly, then make no mistake, you are being very bold, so give yourself a pat on the back. The sad news is that most people will never take the time to learn this stuff and make this brave decision.

Remember: Fortune favours the bold!
You will be rewarded for your efforts.

The one big mistake many books and alkaline diet websites make is in defining acidic and alkaline foods. Many of them class foods as acidic or alkaline based upon their pH in physical form, not on the 'ash' that's produced in the body after it has been metabolized (its correct definition).

This creates confusion and I get emails every week from people who sincerely want to make positive health and nutritional changes, but are simply confused by the conflicting information about the alkaline diet – predominantly regarding which fruits are acidic and alkaline, and whether they should be eaten sparingly or liberally. I can tell you that fruit should most definitely be eaten liberally *but* it should be eaten on its own or before other foods. Ideally you should not eat for at least 2 hours before you eat fruit – otherwise it will ferment on top of other foods and can become acidifying.

This discrepancy in messages from alkaline diet proponents is unhelpful, because the last thing you need when summoning up the courage and discipline to try a new eating regime is to be given conflicting information.

The final piece of 'bad news' I have for you is about the complexity of the alkaline diet. In principle the alkaline diet is very simple: eat alkaline foods and avoid acidic ones. Therefore once you know which is which, surely it's easy? Well, yes, it should be, but many books tend to overcomplicate matters. They talk on about 'colloidal silver supplements' and 'electrical grounding' and say that you need to buy a sprouter, a dehydrator, a masticating juicer and a whole host of other stuff.

Whilst all of this is sound information, it's like trying to run before you can walk. You need to apply the basic principles of drinking lots of water and eliminating smoking, alcohol, refined fats and processed foods *before* you go into the finer details of one alkaline supplement or another. For example – there's no reason to start sprouting your own greens if you are still drinking fizzy sodas and eating lots of junk foods.

It's about addressing the biggest issues first, and the biggest issues for a lot of people, when starting on the path into alkaline health, involve getting more exercise and better sleep, eating enough plant carbohydrates, drinking more pure water, reducing stress and eliminating harmful toxins from their diet. Once those things have been satisfied then you might want to move on to 'Alkaline Diet 202' and beyond. Trying to do everything from the outset can be too overwhelming and complicated, and won't be sustainable long-term because it's too much of a shock – both physically and mentally.

That's why I wrote *The Alkaline 5 Diet* – this book presents a very simple way to eat five meals per day that ensure you are alkalizing your body whilst eating satisfying, simple, delicious meals with foods that are easily available to everyone.

With help from thousands of website subscribers and clients, with all their questions, anecdotes, feedback and experiences, I have come up with a simple Framework for Optimum Health and Healing comprising seven things that will help you achieve your supreme health through the alkaline diet. You'll discover all of this in the following chapters of this book, but the seven elements essential to great health are summarized below:

1. Sunlight and deep oxygenation

2. Pure hydration

3. Sleep and balancing rest

4. Living alkaline foods

5. Eliminating acidic toxins

6. Movement and posture

7. Positive mindset and emotions

Who wins and who loses?

Just like wealth creation, health creation requires us to learn and engage; and furthermore to stop doing the things that unsuccessful people do.

Simply put: people who are successful in pursuing good health tend to eat alkaline foods whilst avoiding acidic toxins, and mindfully engage in lifestyle activities that promote success in this area. People who are unsuccessful in the pursuit of good health live by a different set of maxims, practices and eating habits, although often they are not too far off the mark.

The winners in this game of health are those who engage and educate themselves correctly and act accordingly. The losers are the people who fail to engage and continue to be brainwashed by the media, pharmaceutical companies and food industry; or are simply complacent about their health, resting on the laurels of outward wellbeing, all the while making withdrawals from the bank account of health without making any significant deposits.

The worst situation is to *think* you're engaged and on the right track with health, but have been taken in by the wrong information. As Stephen Covey said, 'If the ladder is not leaning against the right wall, every step we take just gets us to the wrong place faster.'

My mission is to make sure that more people's ladders are firmly against the right wall, where climbing will lead to health, not disease. After all, most of us sincerely want to be healthy and try our best for our families and ourselves. What a tragedy it is that simply as a result of not having the correct information, these efforts are in vain and can lead to disease, despite our best efforts.

Chapter 3

My Health Journey

My health and life journey, as for so many of us, has not been a straight path, but has been made all the more rich and rewarding for having its rolling hills, turns, chicanes and divots. But perhaps I should start by saying that I love food. I am very attuned to my senses and love to experience great sensory pleasures: to look at beautiful things, to hear sublime music, to smell lovely aromas, to experience how dancing and running feels in my body and to eat delicious foods.

Back in my teenage years, the conversation at my all-girls' high school always seemed to be focused on looks, body shape, boys, attractiveness, clothes and generally being judged on how thin and pretty or not we all were. In response I sought comfort in food and developed quite a womanly shape by the time I'd reached 16. I hated it. I disliked all the attention on aesthetics from the girls at school, and new attention from boys, and I felt awkward and out of place much of the time. I just wanted to study and listen to classical music. So I started wearing baggy clothes to hide my figure, avoided socializing and spent more time at home, eating to hide my emotional pain. I also began smoking and drinking.

I became more and more self-conscious, more and more withdrawn and developed more and more unhealthy habits and associations with food, weight and esteem. I enjoyed exercise, particularly swimming, but was so self-conscious that I would only visit the swimming pool late at night when no one else was there.

University wake-up call

At 18 I left home and went to study law at Birmingham University. Thrown into living with 300 other people in a large shared hall of residence was a bit of a shock. I was used to working hard at school, but now partying every day rather than study seemed to be the order of the day. The way I ate changed too, as the catering team's idea of nutrition was fried bacon, eggs, sausages and toast for breakfast and something equally fried and grease-laden for dinner – and everything came with fries.

The result? I spent the first year at university feeling rather inebriated and with an overriding feeling of tiredness and lethargy.

Looking back now, it is obvious why I felt so lacklustre most of the time – alcohol, a poor diet, smoking, not feeling sure of myself and the new situation at university – but at the time I really could not understand why I felt like that and had no energy.

Then I got the wake-up call.

I woke up one weekday at around noon after a heavy night out and noticed that I had developed an itchy, blotchy red rash on my legs. I had never seen anything like it so decided to visit the doctor. After a quick examination, he told me, quite nonchalantly, that I had alcohol poisoning.

Alcohol poisoning! Isn't that what alcoholics get? Just 19 years old and I had poisoned my precious body. I knew I had let my body and myself down. In that moment, I decided things had to change.

Turning things around

I immediately made a positive lifestyle change by joining the local gym and going three times a week. I felt terribly self-conscious at first, but was determined not to let my fear stop me. Then I set myself a goal of being able to run one mile. It took me a couple of weeks because I had really become quite unfit and obviously unhealthy, but I did it and managed to run one mile in around 11 minutes. I felt a real sense of achievement and really good about myself for the first time in a while.

Then I set a target to run that one mile faster; I got it down to 10 minutes.

Then I thought, what if I could run two miles? So I started working up towards this, then three miles and even four.

I was on a roll now. I was starting to get fit and became known at the gym as 'the runner'. A runner? Me? I guess so. They say that the power moves to those that 'do'. I was definitely 'doing' running, so I guess I *was* a runner. Wonderful!

My new exercise regime, my new sense of identity and new self-confidence meant that I had also lost weight; I felt more energetic and happy. All of this gave me the momentum I needed to stop partying so much and to start eating a healthier diet. So I stopped eating the stodgy canteen food and bought my own.

The next stage was to ditch smoking and really start taking nutrition more seriously – which I did when I left uni at 21 and moved back home to Devon. I also got two jobs – I didn't much like the thought of working nine to five.

My first and 'proper' job was working part-time at the local university managing and writing legal policies and reports. My other job was in telesales, working every evening. Having these two jobs allowed me some flexible working habits and time to do my own research, so I started researching health, fitness, nutrition and psychology.

I'd had a taste of success with my exercise regime and wanted to make more progress. Health and fitness intrigued me and I wanted to find out as much as I could about living a great and healthy life.

Encouragement and momentum

My gym training was continuing well and I was now running five or more miles on the treadmill and had started doing some martial arts, Muay Thai boxing and karate, and enjoyed the discipline and challenge of them.

One day Naso, a personal trainer at my YMCA gym, approached me and asked if I was running our local half-marathon. 'No,' I replied. I hadn't even considered it.

She observed that I had been training hard and emphatically encouraged me to apply, in her enthusiastic Greek accent, saying that I'd love it and would do very well. I had never experienced this kind of encouragement in any sport before and it was a novel feeling to be told I'd be really good at something sporty.

I was apprehensive, too. After all, I had been running 5 or so miles, but a half marathon is 13 miles. However, Naso's encouragement had inspired me; I began training to run longer distances and in the end managed a reasonable beginner's time of 2 hours 20 minutes.

It was very physically demanding for me at that time. At one point I thought my lungs were on fire, but I loved the feeling of achievement and the immense tiredness and aching that I got after finishing. It was the kind of tiredness that said, 'I've worked really hard and deserve a lovely rest.' My muscles purred with a contented ache of exertion that we should put our bodies through every now and again, in my view.

That was it; I was sold. I had been bitten by the bug of running endurance races and ran lots of other half-marathons, triathlons, cross country, 10K, trail and other races in the UK and overseas.

I was also reading a lot of inspiring books and quotations at that time and decided that it was time to give a full marathon a go.

The marathons

In December 2003 I decided to start training for the Paris Marathon and began training with my local running group, The Trotters. A veteran runner gave me some advice and told me that as a young first-time marathoner, I should take it easy and walk a few miles so I didn't burn out or hit the wall. So that's what I did and ran it in 4 hours 48 minutes, but I felt I had undersold myself and could have run a quicker time.

So I decided that I would run the race again next year – *my* way.

I found a great running partner, Mike, from my local gym, and we got down to some serious training. One of our favourite training runs was on Dartmoor around a reservoir. The course was four miles and we worked up to running three times around, four times around and eventually five times around – 20 miles.

We were preparing well, plus I had made some great dietary changes – I was eating huge amounts of fresh raw vegetables and fruits each day, as well as some grains, such as rice and quinoa, and that was pretty much it. I was following the alkaline diet intuitively and it was giving me loads of energy and aiding a very quick recovery from intense exercise sessions. I felt fantastic!

The feeling when I crossed the finish line on race-day was unbelievable. Coming down the last stretch, I ran as fast as I could. I always finish a race strong and try my best to sprint. I crossed the line and felt such euphoria! It was like a party suddenly started in my head: I had been so mentally constrained and focused for the last 4 hours that it was such a mental release to finish and my mind went wild. So happy and joyous!

I looked at my watch… 3 hours 48 minutes. I had achieved my goal and knocked a *whole hour* off my previous time. That is a great memory for me.

I truly believe that my clean, alkaline diet was a huge contributing factor in my race success. It certainly gave me loads of energy and fast recovery times, as well as mental clarity and concentration; and I never experienced cramps or injuries, despite pushing myself hard on a daily basis.

My work

As you can imagine, I was now completely sold on a healthy lifestyle and the joy it could bring. As well as running and going to the gym, I was out dancing each week, enjoying the feelings of supreme fitness and health and marvelling at the wonders of the human body. I now knew that I wanted to work in health and thought, *What better place to work than the health service?*

Little did I know….

I applied for a position as medical research manager and got it. My job was to review all of the medical research proposals that were put forward by doctors, surgeons, consultants, nurses and other health practitioners, and to vet them against legal and ethical standards of safety, viability and soundness, as well as expense and funding.

In short, my boss and I, along with a medical ethics committee, had the final say on whether a research proposal was given the go-ahead to be turned into a full-blown clinical research trial.

The job was fascinating: an insider's view on the latest double-blind randomized diabetes drug trials, cancer research and schizophrenia studies; having the responsibility of ensuring patient safety and ethics; and liaising with some brilliant researchers and medical professionals. I was also responsible for some pretty big things: I organized and chaired a large health research seminar and prepared the annual research report that went to the government, but something began to bother me.

The first thing that hit me early on was that most of the so-called medical experts were often obese and looked positively unhealthy. I mused to myself about this phenomenon: would a criminal be allowed to serve in the police force (OK, don't answer that one). Would a person who could not drive be allowed to work as a driving instructor?

You could argue that you don't need to be a good player to be able to coach, but in order to coach any sport you *must* be able to play at least adequately, if not at a high level.

The second, and much more disturbing, thing I noticed was a common theme in the research proposals that were given the go-ahead and the ones that were refused. The ones that passed through easily and smoothly, with little challenge to aspects such as likelihood of cure of condition, were the ones that required long-term medication, which would not actually cure but rather *manage* the disease or condition – such as diabetes drugs.

The ones that were repeatedly refused were the ones that involved so-called wacky new concepts, such as using vegetables and fruits to cure disease. There was one doctor in particular I recall who had conducted extensive research and he wanted to get medical ethics approval in order to roll it out on a larger scale. He claimed that he had used large volumes of fresh vegetables in patients' diets to slow down the growth of cancer and in some cases, reverse it.

This kind of study really interested me and I was keen for it to be given the go-ahead. I had read some of Ann Wigmore's work about how she had used organic veg and wheatgrass juice in the sixties at her Hippocrates Health Institute in the USA to cure terminally ill patients. So I didn't think this was 'wacky' at all, it made utter sense to me. Yet the doctor who put forward his proposal in this area was ousted from his position and became the joke of the medical research community.

It dawned on me that it was the pharmaceutical companies that provided most of the medical research funding (which I now had intimate knowledge of). If you haven't guessed it already, here's the connection… it took a while for the penny to really drop for me, apologies if you've made the connection already:

The pharma companies have a vested, and hugely profitable, interest in keeping people on drugs for years and years. This is the perfect type of disease management from their perspective. They are not concerned with finding a real cure (end of drug-taking and money); they are not concerned with managing and curing illness by natural means (no money at all for them), so they tend only to fund and pass policies (yes, pharma companies have a massive impact and say in medical research policy formulation) that support *their* best interests (money), *not* yours and mine (to be free from disease and in good health).

I remember thinking that I had joined the health service to do exactly that – serve health. By this time I knew that this job would *never* allow me truly to do that and I was, in fact, working for the ill-health service. There was no emphasis on what it meant to be really healthy: happy, energetic, positive, strong and free from disease, not managing it with expensive potions with all their outrageous side effects.

So when my boss offered to renew my contract and promote me to a higher level, with a significant pay rise, I politely declined the renewal and left the job shortly afterwards.

My website

In 2008, I went to Anthony Robbins' legendary 'Unleash the Power Within' seminar. Tony is just an absolute powerhouse of energy and the four-day mammoth event in London that I attended with 12,000 other people was mind-blowing to say the least.

The last day of the event was all about vitality and health and he mentioned this dietary protocol called the 'alkaline diet' – the what? I had never heard this name before and I was intrigued. As the day went on and we were given a detailed description, explanation of the benefits and plan for following the alkaline diet, I realized that this was the diet I had been following of my own accord and getting great results with for years.

A year later, I set up my website, Alkaline Diet Health Tips, and began writing articles and recipe books centred on a fruit-and-vegetable-based diet.

Today, I have many thousands of subscribers to my website, from more than 50 different countries, and am privileged to receive emails and feedback every day of the week from people sharing their experiences and successes with both my own materials and resources and the alkaline, vegan and raw food diets in general.

> *Thanks for your website articles. Earlier this year my two-year-old son Ben was diagnosed with type 1 diabetes. We have since put him on a total raw food alkaline diet and have been learning about a more alkaline diet for our whole family. I am happy to say that Ben's diabetes seems to be reversing, in that he needs very little injected insulin, if any, and that his blood sugar levels are staying within a healthy, normal range. What seemed to be a great discouragement for us has turned out to be a blessing for us, as this has led us all to take a closer look at the quality of food that we prepare and eat. Thanks, and keep up the good work! –* ELIDAD

Since setting up my site, I have researched more, interviewed many other experts, surveyed, questioned and interacted with my subscribers and customers about their experiences and gained a whole new level of understanding; and their stories, along with all the information and research I've gathered, is what you'll find in the coming chapters of this book.

*I have been living the alkaline lifestyle since 2006. I am
47 years old and feel like a teenager – very strong and
healthy. I felt sick and tired six years ago, now my cancer
has been eradicated!* – FAUSTO

Where I am now

Since my 3:48 Paris Marathon, I have gone on to run many
more endurance races and triathlons. Between 2013 and 2014,
I ran 12 marathon distances and races and one ultra-marathon
of 32 miles across hilly moors. I know it's my diet and lifestyle
that have allowed me to live energetically and vibrantly and
keep my fitness and exercise levels to a very high standard
since 2002.

Here are the objective facts of what I've attained on the
Alkaline 5 Diet:

◆ I am very lean, fit and flexible, and have good muscle
tone.

◆ My skin and hair look better than when I was 17 years old
and I am regularly told that I look radiant and 10 years
younger than my actual age.

◆ I have sustained energy throughout the day, every day. I
do not drink coffee or take any other stimulants.

◆ I take no pharmaceutical or other drugs whatsoever.

◆ I have the mental resilience and focus to run my business
and speak at events as well as live a varied life of
travelling, singing in a philharmonic choir, Latin dancing
and various sports such as surfing and cycling, as well as
running.

I am happy; I love to learn new things; and have great relationships with positive people around me. It's been a long path to get to where I am today and I want to help you achieve similarly great health too, not necessarily to run marathons, but for whatever motivates you and brings you joy.

Encouragement makes all the difference; just as I was encouraged back in my early twenties by a few loving people, I wish to encourage you that you are *destined* for supreme health and to live your best life EVER.

So let's make a start, shall we?

Part I
The Framework for Supreme Health, Healing and Vitality

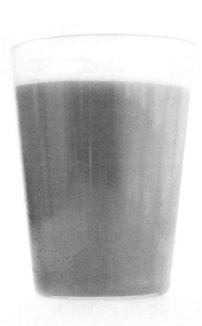

Introduction

Essential Elements for Health

I created the Framework for Optimum Health and Healing to make it easy to understand and follow the seven distinctive and essential elements for achieving superb health through nutrition and lifestyle practice.

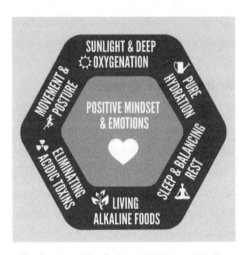

The Framework for Optimum Health and Healing

Let's look at each one briefly, before we go into greater depth in the next chapters.

1. Sunlight and deep oxygenation

Of course, getting oxygen through breathing is the number one most important necessity in our lives. However, many of us are breathing on a very superficial level, taking shallow breaths throughout most of the day. It is vitally important to get proper, effective oxygenation; and this is achieved by mindful deep breathing and by aerobic exercise. We will look at some effective breathing techniques and some great ways to get your body moving for optimum oxygenation.

2. Pure hydration

Most people know the benefits of drinking lots of fresh, clean pure water throughout the day, but not all water is made equal. Whether it is chlorine and fluoride in your tap water or plastic chemicals in bottled waters, the water we are drinking may not actually be optimal for our health, so we are going to look at the options for getting the best water possible for super-clean hydration, including the ins and outs of alkaline water.

3. Sleep and balancing rest

Not getting enough good-quality sleep and rest has the tendency to put all other aspects of our lives out of kilter. Often dietary problems can arise from being deprived of sleep, making us reach for the wrong types of foods and elevating our levels of cortisol and stress hormones – which encourages weight gain. This is an aspect of health that many people don't take seriously, while knowing how important it is to get proper sleep. So let me ask you, are you consistently getting 8–10 hours of sleep and rest per night?

4. Living alkaline foods

Eating living, raw foods, such as leafy green vegetables, fruits and sprouted seeds, is your pathway to excellent health. The ideal balance is around 70 per cent raw plant-based foods and 30 per cent cooked (more acidic) foods by calories, which can come from a number of different sources, depending on your preference, and still allows for 'treat' foods.

The alkalizing effects of a raw plant-based diet are phenomenal and play a huge part in our overall vitality and health. Alkalizing the body helps to guard against disease and illness and contributes massively to achieving both sustained high energy and a calm state of mind.

Many people who have a high proportion of living alkaline foods in their diet claim that it helps change all areas of their life in a very positive way: It's not just about the food, it's about an elevated state of being.

5. Eliminating acidic toxins

We are constantly bombarded with toxins and poisons; it's just a fact of modern living. However, there are many toxins that we can avoid and eliminate from our lives when we have the right information to make some intelligent lifestyle switches. For example, aluminium in antiperspirant deodorants and other beauty products has been linked with serious health conditions, such as Alzheimer's disease,[1] while parabens, found in beauty products like shampoos, conditioners and shower gels, have been linked to cancer.[2] Switching to more natural products is not particularly onerous or inconvenient, but could make a massive difference to your long-term health.

6. Movement and posture

Since most of us live in a culture where sedentary office jobs, sitting down a lot of the time and driving a car is the norm, it can be easy to neglect the fact that we are designed to move on a regular basis, just like our animal friends. Spending a good proportion of your day standing up, and moving and maintaining good posture whilst sitting down can have an immediate and very positive effect on your health and wellbeing. Simple habits, such as taking regular breaks throughout the day and stretching, can help with both of these things.

7. Positive mindset and emotions

Cultivating a positive and upbeat mindset by focusing on positive thoughts and emotions, and not dwelling on negative ones, plays a huge part in your wellbeing and health. You could be eating all the right things, exercising, taking superfoods, drinking plenty of water… but if you are stressed, cynical or negative then you simply won't achieve the great health that is possible for you.

Many people are surprised to learn (or unwilling to accept) that a positive mindset and happiness are *not* dependent on outside circumstances – e.g., I am happy when someone is nice to me and unhappy when someone is nasty to me. We are the masters of our emotions and success in life comes from *choosing* happiness and gratitude, not the other way around. We will look at some very definite ways to cultivate a superior mindset.

Let's now go into each of the seven principles of the Framework for Optimum Health and Healing in more depth in the next chapters.

My arthritis plagued me for years; every little thing gave me pain in my hands. I thought I'd try the alkaline diet as I'd heard so many good things about it. After only a week I was able to open jars without any pain, which I hadn't been able to do for years. That was the first thing I noticed. My health has just got better and better since then and I'm now living pain-free and off any medication. It feels like a new lease of life. I am so grateful. – MATTHEW

Chapter 4

A Big Breath of Fresh Air: Deep Oxygenation

What do running, smelling flowers, being near water and singing all have in common?

They all increase oxygenation in the body.

Perhaps running is the most obvious example because our heart rate elevates and we breathe more deeply to get oxygen pumping around our bodies to feed our muscles. Exercise forces us to breathe much more deeply. Singing requires deep and controlled diaphragm breathing and is a great way to oxygenate your whole body. Being a singer in various bands and choirs for many years, I can definitely attest to not only the 'good for the soul' benefits of singing, but also those for physical wellbeing.

The importance of deep oxygenation

Quite simply, our levels of health are directly related to our levels of energy. Energy is created at a cellular level in our bodies and cells need a lot of oxygen in order to create the ATP (Adenosine Triphosphate),[1] which fuels us.

Without adequate oxygen, we cannot produce ATP and without ATP we would die. That is why we can only hold our breath for a very short period of time before we are in deep trouble. Healthy cells in our bodies are aerobic and oxygen is right up there as the body's most important nutrient.

In 1931, Nobel Prize winner Otto Warburg made a connection between oxygen and cancer.[2] He discovered that the number one cause of cancer was a lack of proper oxygenation in the cellular environment. He found that cancer cells thrive in an oxygen-deprived environment and cannot live in an oxygen-rich one. Warburg also made a connection between the body's pH and degenerative disease (including cancer). He believed that a higher pH (i.e. alkaline cells) gave rise to higher oxygen in the cells and guarded against disease.

Furthermore, deep breathing stimulates the body's lymphatic system. Unlike our blood system, our lymph system doesn't have a pump (the heart pumps the blood) and needs to be activated by movement and deep breathing.

Applying the principle of deep oxygenation

Here follow some great ways to oxygenate your body and provide a good flow of oxygen to your cells. In all the following suggestions, remember that it's also important to be mindful of your posture, because hunching over when sitting or standing leads to shallow breathing.

Deep diaphragm breathing

It's good to get into the habit of doing ten or so deep belly breaths a few times per day. This expands your diaphragm muscle and the alveoli air pockets in your lungs, which in turn de-stresses you and stimulates your lymph system instantly.

The correct practice is to breathe air deep into your lower abdomen, without raising your shoulders. Your belly should expand and then, when you breathe out, it should be like squeezing a plastic bottle full of water, squeezing the air out of your lungs.

A great rhythm to get into with your deep breathing is to breathe in for a count of four, hold your breath for a count of eight (this gives your cells a chance to dump excess carbon dioxide and other waste materials into your oxygenated blood) and then breathe out steadily for a count of 16 (expelling the toxins). So the ratio is 1:2:4 – breathe in for four, hold for eight, and then out for 16.

You may need to build up to doing this because it requires a degree of both control and fitness, and you may find you feel light-headed at first because your body's not used to such a hit of oxygen. If this is the case, start off with a ratio of 1:1:2 – breathe in for four, hold for four, and then out for eight.

Do a set of 10 of these breathing exercises once or twice a day; they are great to do first thing in the morning.

Aerobic exercise

Any exercise that raises your heart rate and gets you breathing harder and faster is a good form of aerobic exercise. Walking, running, cycling, rowing, badminton, tennis, skating, swimming, dancing, boxing, surfing, rebounding; the list is endless. Pick an activity or combination of activities that you enjoy and is sustainable for you.

Consistency is the key here. It's no good doing something aerobically beneficial that you hate and then only doing it once a month. It's better to find something as hard or as gentle as suits you, but then sticking with it over the long term. Aim for at least 30 minutes, three times per week, but preferably five times per week or, better still, every day.

So, as an example, you could walk briskly for 30 minutes first thing on Monday, Wednesday and Friday mornings, cycle on Tuesday evenings, swim for 30 minutes on Thursday evening and do a jive or street-dance class on Friday evening.

🌿 Alkaline-delicious tip 🌿

Before you start any exercise regime it is recommended that you seek advice from your medical professional.

🌿🌿

Singing

Having a good old warble (or playing any kind of blowing, wind or brass instrument) is great for deeply oxygenating your body. Typically – and especially if you have learned breathing technique for singing – you take quick, diaphragm in-breaths followed by slow, controlled and sustained out-breaths to sing the notes. This is a great way to make deep, effective breathing fun and enjoyable!

So put on the radio or your favourite CD and sing along for about 10 minutes every day.

The benefits of applying this principle

When you start incorporating some, or hopefully all, of the deep oxygenation practices in your life, you will experience some distinct benefits, including:

- Feeling more relaxed, centred and calm, and less stressed

- More effective immune system, resulting in fewer minor and major illnesses

- Stronger core abdominal muscles and a flatter stomach

- Improved skin tone and colour

- Fewer back, neck and joint aches and pains

- Improved flexibility

Chapter 5

Plump Your Cells, Lubricate Your Brain

Next to oxygen, water is the most essential substance for life, and makes up 80 per cent of our cells, organs and, therefore, whole body.

Hydration is about drinking the correct amount of pure clean water each day to meet your individual body's needs. The amount of water required varies from person to person and is dependent largely on your weight, activity levels and the climate you live in. For example, a tall, heavy, muscular man who works out a lot and lives in a hot country will require a lot more water than a small-framed woman who works in an office and is not particularly active.

That said, many people are chronically dehydrated,[1-2] regardless of any differing factors that affect their hydration needs. A small, inactive woman still requires at least 2 litres (3½ pints) of water each day. A muscular, very active man probably needs more like 4–5 litres (7–8¾ pints) each day.

In my experience, many people say that they drink a lot of water (it's the first thing I ask clients when they say they are tired, ill, overweight etc.), but when probed they often admit that they are not really sure if they are drinking 2 litres (3½ pints) or more *every* day, consistently. Coffee and tea *do not* count as water. Fruit drinks *do not* count as water. Sodas, alcohol or any other drink *apart* from pure water do NOT count as water![3]

To me it seems strange that so many people have an aversion to drinking water. Don't be one of those people who make it harder than it needs to be. Just do it! Drinking water is beautiful. It's one of the kindest, most lovely things you can do for your body and mind.

The importance of pure hydration

We use up and lose water in many bodily functions and processes so we need to replenish our water levels constantly in order to stay properly hydrated. Everything that happens in our bodies requires water – respiration, digestion, urination, sweating, anabolic and catabolic processes (building up and breaking down of tissue, fat and muscle) – and all of these processes dehydrate us.

If we all ate bountiful amounts of fresh vegetables and fruits, which can constitute as much as 90 per cent water, our need to drink water in order to keep hydrated would be much less. But since most of us don't do this, we do need to drink lots of water – enough water, every day.

✾ Alkaline-delicious tip ✾

Every cell in your body needs to be well hydrated at all times in order to thrive. Cells need to be like plump grapes, rather than dried prunes. Plus, if you've ever struggled with weight loss, you should know that good hydration is one of the best ways to regulate your appetite, lose weight and keep it off over the long term.[4]

Our bodies can operate on below-par levels of water because they are miraculous and highly adaptable super-machines, but there is a high price to pay: below-par mental and physical health and performance. The first thing to be compromised is mental clarity and your ability to eliminate waste, and therefore constipation is a big indicator of dehydration. Some erroneous definitions of constipation state that it is having fewer than three bowel movements per week. I believe this is in fact severe constipation.

Dehydration is the root cause of and exacerbates many diseases.[4,5]

Applying the principle of pure hydration

The key to pure hydration is based around three things:

1. Quantity

2. Quality

3. Regularity

Quality

Not all water is created equal. Tap water almost always contains lots of toxins and heavy metals that are not good for us and can be very dangerous to health, for example chlorine and fluorine compounds.[6]

In many countries it is advised not to drink tap water, but certainly also if you live in the UK or USA, the quality of water is quite poor – containing all sorts of chemicals that often pass water quality tests because they are tasteless and odourless. There are literally thousands of harmful pollutants that go unidentified and undetected in tap water.[7–9]

The water in many areas of the UK contains fluoride and, despite what dentists and the media will have us believe, fluoride is not good for your teeth. Man-made fluoride, if taken in excess quantities, can actually lead to fluorosis, a condition marked by stained and weakened cavity-filled teeth. Notably, in Europe and US communities where there is no water fluoridation, the population suffer fewer cavities than in fluoridated US communities.

Even worse, fluoride is toxic for our health and can result in hyperactivity and/or lethargy, arthritis, lowered thyroid function, lowered IQ, dementia, disrupted immune system, genetic damage, cell death, cancers, deactivated essential enzymes and reduced lifespan.[10]

You may wonder why fluoride is put into our water and advocated by dentists. I have often wondered this and explanations can range from ignorance to profit to conspiracy. Suffice to say that we need to be vigilant ourselves in ensuring that we are not taking in fluoride through the water we drink.

Therefore, drinking acidic tap water is out – unless you are happy to live with below-par health. Bottled mineral water may taste better than tap water but, in many cases, it still contains impurities and can often contain chemicals and oestrogens from the plastic bottles that it is stored in. Glass bottles are a better option.

We need to be drinking pure water that is above pH7 because drinking alkaline water is one of the fastest and most effective ways of restoring your body's acid–alkaline balance. Pure water that has not been treated with harsh chemicals and toxins is naturally oxygenated and slightly alkaline. Since it is near impossible to find, other than very pure spring water, it is best to 'make' your own alkaline water, and that can be achieved in a number of ways.

1. Water ionizers

These machines fix to your standard taps (faucets) or plumbing and produce alkaline water by running it over positive and negative electrodes, which first filters then ionizes the incoming water.

Ionizers typically filter out inorganic and organic chemicals, lead and many other heavy metals, pesticides, trihalomethanes and volatile organic chemicals (e.g., chloroform and radon gas), detergents, asbestos, some viruses and pollens. They don't, however, filter out the minerals, which are soluble in water, and this is a benefit. Unlike distillers or reverse osmosis (RO) devices, water ionizers leave in all of the minerals that your body requires for proper functioning. You are left with nothing but clean, mineralized water, which is ready for the ionization process.

During ionization, the soluble minerals are attracted to either the positive electrode or the negative one, depending on their own electrical energy. When this happens, the water separates into alkaline and acid streams.

The alkaline water is used for drinking, while the acid water can be used for washing, heating, feeding plants and disinfecting. The great benefit here is that harmful minerals (and mineral compounds such as fluoride) polarize and flow out with the acidic water while the positive minerals flow out with the alkaline, leaving you with healthy, ionized drinking water.

Water ionizers can be either countertop or under-sink units and they are an expensive investment. Over a lifetime, of course, they are relatively low maintenance and a cost-effective way of creating pure water. The filters do need to be replaced every six to twelve months, dependent on volume usage, but are relatively inexpensive.

Considering that we need large quantities of water every day of our life and drinking high-quality water has the potential to affect every other area of our life positively – from sleep to concentration to weight regulation to teeth and bone health – I'd say installing an water ionizer is a very worthy investment in the big picture of things.

2. Water Distillers

Distilled water is contentious: many scientists and health experts advocate it as the best overall option for consumption while others say that it is not good for health at all. Water is distilled when it is heated up until it turns to steam and then condenses back into liquid water. By its nature, distilled water contains no impurities or minerals and its pH is very close to neutral. However, you do not get the benefits of any alkaline minerals so it is recommended that distilled water is used in conjunction with pH drops. There is also potential concern with distilled water that is worth mentioning.

Research conducted by the Swiss chemist and Nobel Prize nominee Dr Paul Kouchakoff in the thirties indicated that only eating cooked food provoked an increase in white blood cell activity (which happens when the body's fights an infection). The 'flash point' of water is considered to be around 77°C (170°F). Some scientists believe that consuming water heated above 77°C (170°F) can promote an increase in white blood cell activity, even if the water is consumed after cooling.[11] Bottled distilled water carries the same dangers as bottled mineral water – the potential for leaching plastics from the container into the water, thereby contaminating it. A home-distillation system overcomes this problem and is relatively inexpensive because it requires little maintenance. However, the water is not available 'on tap' because it takes a few hours to produce.

3. Reverse osmosis water (RO) machines

The reverse osmosis process uses a semi-permeable membrane to remove up to 99 per cent of impurities and chemicals, such as chloride, fluoride, lead, iron, nitrate, magnesium, copper, sodium, viruses, arsenic, oestrogen and bacteria, using only water pressure.

RO machines are considerably cheaper than ionizers initially; however, the membranes need to be replaced fairly often, in comparison to ionizer filters (approximately every six months). Filters are relatively inexpensive, but good maintenance of your RO machine is necessary, or else the machine can let mould, bacteria and other contaminants through the membrane.

Also, as with distillers, it takes a while to produce the water and it contains no alkaline minerals, so is not properly alkaline-balanced. It is therefore recommended that RO water be used in conjunction with pH drops or a mineral filter.

4. Alkaline Water Jugs and Filter Jugs

These are better options than tap water and certainly far cheaper than ionizers or RO machines; however, they do not have the ability to completely filter out volatile organic compounds (VOCs), hormones and pharmaceuticals. Also, they are smaller in size and can only filter a jug at a time. I'd say this is a good interim choice before getting one of the other better options listed above.

5. pH drops

Adding pH drops, which contain alkaline compounds such as hydrogen peroxide, to water is a relatively cheap way to alkalize your water. However, none of the water's chemicals and pollutants are filtered out, so it's only as good as the quality of the original tap water in essence, but with a bit of an alkaline boost. Therefore, pH drops are best used with distilled or RO water.

6. Adding alkaline ingredients to drinking water

Adding the juice of a whole, freshly squeezed lemon or lime to your drinking water gives it an alkaline boost. Lemons and limes are alkalizing to your body (yes, they're acidic in their physical form, but as they are metabolized by your body, they leave alkaline minerals). Simple but effective. Another way is to add green powders – such as wheatgrass juice powder.

As with pH drops, it is still recommended that you use a distiller, RO machine or ionizer, as well as adding alkaline ingredients, to ensure the water is pure.

7. Bottled water

Only buy water labelled 'mineral water' and preferably in glass bottles, as other waters such as 'spring' or 'table' are often no more than glorified tap water. Bottled water is better than tap water, but more expensive than buying an ionizer, distiller or RO machine in the long term.

How much water should you drink?

The rule of thumb is that you should drink 1 litre (1¾ pints) of water per 18kgs (40lbs) of body weight. If you are very inactive then you can decrease this by around 30 per cent.

Therefore, if you weigh 63.5kgs (140lbs) you would require 3.5 litres (6 pints) of water per day (or 2.5 litres/4½ pints if you're inactive). This is greatly more than the recommended six to eight glasses per day.

To ensure you get your full daily requirements, fill a 2-litre (3½-pint) bottle and work your way through it during the day. If you weigh 72.5kgs (160lbs) then you would need to fill your 2-litre (3½-pint) bottle twice to get your recommended 4 litres (7 pints). This takes away the thinking and makes it easy. Just like setting up a direct debit to deposit money straight from your bank account to your savings account each month.

Be careful not to drink *too* much water, as this is dangerous and can lead to a condition called hypernatremia (water intoxication). You'd have to drink many litres (pints) though to upset your electrolyte balance; dehydration is much more likely than hypernatremia – just don't zealously overdo the water.

Drinking water throughout the day

Drink regularly throughout the day – every 30 minutes is ideal. It is much better to drink smaller amounts consistently and regularly all day long than to drink 2 litres (3½ pints) in one go. That said, it's great to drink ½ a litre (18fl oz) or 1 litre (1¾ pints) of water first thing in the morning upon waking, since you'll be dehydrated from sleeping.

It is also best to drink water before and between meals, not with or after meals, so that your digestive enzymes are not diluted when eating, as this can impair the digestive and absorption processes.

The benefits of applying this principle

Here are the main signs to indicate that you are drinking enough water:

♦ Clear and odourless urine

♦ Urinating at least 8–10 times per day

♦ Steady energy levels

♦ Soft skin

♦ Relatively odour-free perspiration

♦ Moist mouth and lips

♦ Regular soft bowel movements with pain-free elimination

In addition, here are a few of the benefits of pure hydration.

♦ Greater energy

♦ Reduces headaches and migraines

♦ Clears skin

♦ Improves sleep

♦ Regulates appetite

♦ Better concentration and brainpower

♦ Prevents disease and illness

♦ Weight loss or regulation – reaching and maintaining your optimum weight

♦ Treats fluid retention

- ♦ Improves muscle tone

- ♦ Relieves constipation

- ♦ Relieves back and joint pain

For a guide to water ionizers and other alkaline water machines and where to buy them, see the Resources section, page 231.

I suffered from fibromyalgia, which was very painful and I was almost disabled. Then I read about alkaline water and the body's pH levels. I bought a water ionizer, which increases the water's alkalinity, and started drinking only that for my water and herbal tea. I drink about 3 litres (5¼ pints) a day. Within four weeks the pain was going away. Within four months, I was completely pain-free. I can't make any claim as to whether it was responsible or not, but I feel like a new person. – STEPHEN

Chapter 6

Dreams Abounding:
Sleep and Balancing Rest

Getting a good night's sleep is so natural and so easy, and yet many of us struggle to go to sleep, stay asleep and get enough.

Sleep quality is inhibited by all manner of factors in our modern age – the advent of electricity being the biggest factor. Artificial lights mean that we can stay awake and active long after sundown, which was once our natural indicator to sleep.

Electricity also means that we are accustomed to watching television in the evening, using computers and other electrical and entertainment devices, socializing and partying, and generally forcing our bodies to be still up and functioning long into the night – past sundown and often much later. Coupled with stimulants such as caffeine and then the need to arise for work, it's no wonder we are sleep-deprived.

Adequate sleep is absolutely, 100 per cent, vitally important for excellent health. You can be fit, eat a great diet, get lots of fresh air and sunshine, but if you are sleep-deprived, you cannot reach your health potential and there is a high price to pay for this deprivation.

The importance of sleep and rest

Sleep is essential to recharge your nervous system – it gives your brain sufficient downtime, making it more efficient during your waking hours.

Your brain is the control centre of your body, and a well-rested brain produces great results throughout your body, mind, emotions and spirit.

When we are sleep-deprived, we are likely to feel on edge and on constant alert. If you have ever had jet lag, you'll know the feeling, and it results in poor concentration, low energy levels and poor dietary choices as we look for something to give us a lift in energy, such as a cup of coffee or a bar of chocolate.

Sleep is the only thing that recharges your batteries and allows your body to properly eliminate waste and toxins. Getting enough sleep and rest also helps build muscle, regenerate your cells and tissue, and break down fat and toxins.

Applying the principle of nourishing sleep and rest

The old saying 'early to bed, early to rise makes you healthy, wealthy and wise' is a truism if ever there was one. There is nothing like going to bed early – around 10 p.m. – then sleeping for 8–10 hours and arising fresh, alert and excited to begin your day.

It's also true that the hours you sleep before midnight count for double in terms of rest. We produce more melatonin between 9 p.m. and midnight than after this time. Melatonin regulates our body's circadian rhythm (sleep/wake cycle) and is an antioxidant. So there is also truth in the phrase 'beauty sleep' –

more melatonin whilst you sleep helps to slow down the ageing process by mopping up free radicals in your body.[1]

Melatonin production, however, is halted by light so it's important to ensure that you sleep in a dark room. It is also vitally important to wind down in the evenings before going to bed: lower the lights and do not watch television before bed. If you like to read before falling asleep, make sure that it's a physical book with a low room light and avoid any backlit electronic devices.

Getting the sleep and rest you need

I have tried all types of sleep regimes and patterns and suffered with insomnia for years in my early twenties. The problem was I was doing all the wrong things without consciously realizing it: going to bed starving hungry after fitness training, having the lights on right up until sleep time, going to bed at irregular hours and late, stimulating my mind by reading business books, checking emails and even doing work! I now sleep well and here's what I recommend for optimum rest.

♦ Start winding down at 9 p.m. Lower the lights and stop engaging in stimulating activities. Go to bed at 10 p.m. (or no later than 11 p.m.) and keep your sleep hours regular.

♦ Do not eat for two hours before you sleep. Instead have a small healthy snack or meal in the evening no later than 8 p.m. if you are very hungry.

♦ Sleep in a very dark room with the window open or on the latch to allow some fresh air in and no lights – no LED clocks, no phone in your bedroom, no TV, no electrical gadgets. The goal is to eliminate electromagnetic frequency (EMF) radiation and stimulants whilst sleeping. You might also want to fit blackout blinds and/or curtains if light pollution from streetlights is an issue.

♦ Turn off your Internet Wi-Fi, as this disrupts sleep greatly. Have an analogue clock in your room if you must have one. Get 8 to 10 or more hours' sleep and wake up naturally.[2]

♦ Keep your bedroom clean and tidy – change your bed covers regularly, dust and vacuum regularly and use natural fibres in your bedding: 100 per cent cotton sheets, down duvet or quilt and a great-quality pocket-sprung mattress are best.

♦ There is evidence to suggest that memory foam mattresses give off harmful chemical vapours that can cause all manner of health problems. From my own experience, I had sleep problems when I had a memory foam mattress and also used to wake up with an overwhelming feeling of needing fresh air. When I saw the research on vapours from memory foam, it really resonated with my experience; I got rid of the mattress immediately and have not had the problems since.[3,4]

♦ Take naps when you can. Animals take naps whenever they feel like it. They don't ask permission, they don't feel guilty; they just do it. So as far as your lifestyle permits, take as much rest as you need whenever you feel like it. Your health will benefit greatly from it.

♦ Your bedroom should be for sleep, lovemaking, prayer and reading only.

We are socially conditioned to stay awake and alert and 'perk ourselves up' with caffeine and stimulants, but why? So we can work longer hours in a job we dislike? Don't get caught up in this social competition of who can get more done and sleep the least; it's a game that will bring you down. Sooner or later, your body will balk against it and force you to rest by becoming ill or injured and then you won't be able to do anything.

I have experienced this myself by doing too much, working too many hours and not getting enough rest, and then all of a sudden suffering a severe back injury that came out of nowhere and put me completely out of action for almost a month – I literally couldn't move or walk for a week and couldn't exercise for much longer. Looking back, this was a blessing in disguise because it forced me to slow down and rest, so I could work and train smarter rather than longer and harder.

✿ Alkaline-delicious tip ✿

There is no badge of honour for having less sleep. So many people think that it's better to have only 5 or 6 hours' sleep per night, rather than 10 or more. This is very naive and a false economy in the long term. When you get 10 hours of sleep per night, your waking capabilities in all areas of life greatly surpass those people who are functioning below par on less sleep.

✿✿✿

The benefits of applying this principle

Here are just a few of the benefits of getting high-quality, high-quantity sleep and rest:

♦ Feeling alive and vital with sustained energy

♦ Feeling less tired during the day

♦ Feeling calmer and more able to cope with life's stresses

♦ Properly balanced hunger mechanism and less likelihood of overeating or emotional eating

♦ Weight loss and muscle gain as your body has proper time for anabolic and catabolic processes

♦ Greater ability to concentrate and focus

♦ Better skin

♦ A leaner waist as less cortisol is produced (and likewise other stress hormones that contribute to abdominal fat retention)

♦ Quicker recovery times between exercise sessions

♦ Greater athletic and strength performance

♦ Feeling happier

♦ Looking and feeling younger

Chapter 7

Live and Let Live:
Living Alkaline Foods

Food and eating is an inescapable reality of our everyday lives and takes up a great deal of time each day. We have to eat every few hours or so and it should be an enjoyable and health-giving activity, but for the vast majority of people in the world it poses some major issues.

In the developing world, the issue is often a dire one, as the prime concern is getting enough food to sustain life, let alone good health. In the Western world it can range from the trivial, such as choosing what to have for lunch, to a complex eating disorder, such as anorexia or morbid obesity, and a spectrum of issues in between.

Food and eating is unlike the previous three principles – oxygenation, hydration and sleep – because these factors are binary in nature; either you get enough sleep, or you don't. Either you're well hydrated and oxygenated, or you're not.

Food is a much more complex subject because there is not just one type of food that we should be eating, and it is not a simple element or singular compound. Instead there is an infinite choice in how we satisfy our need for fuel via the consumption of food and it is influenced by many external factors.

Our daily food choices are a delicate art and science that pose minefields at every juncture, unless we're highly attuned to our body's needs and well informed about good and bad dietary practices. What's more, some strength of character is required, if we are to rise above all the social/societal norms and conditioning around food and eat *only* for the purpose of fuelling our bodies to support a vibrant life.

Let me ask you this: Who do you know who ONLY eats healthy foods and in moderation – eating when hungry and stopping before full? A person who doesn't eat because it is sociable to do so, or because a family member has cooked for them, or because they are feeling bored and food provides temporary amusement… but rather because they are depleted of energy and need to eat at that particular moment?

I doubt you can name anyone. Neither can I, although I know a handful of people who come close to this – but they are world experts in diet and nutrition, and have been practising and teaching nutrition for decades; they're not your average Joe.

So if, at the moment, you are aware that your diet and eating practices are less than optimal, it's OK, and for the most part it's not your fault. However it *is* your responsibility to make some positive and courageous changes to reach your physical, mental and emotional optimum via your food choices.

The brilliant news is that the Alkaline 5 Diet gives you a way to eat both healthfully and deliciously at the same time, because I love food and so I designed A5D to meet five specific criteria, as follows:

1. Simple

2. Satisfying

3. Super-healthy

4. Sustainable

5. Systematized

We'll look at the principles of the Alkaline 5 Diet and foods we can eat in Part II, but for now here is a list of just some of the factors that can have very pervasive influences on our ability to decide what we eat and when:

♦ Food industry advertising and indoctrination

♦ Supermarket and grocery store layout and offerings

♦ TV commercials

♦ Diet industry books and marketing

♦ Diet industry contradictions

♦ Contradictions about what is best to eat leading to confusion, inaction and apathy

♦ Dairy industry funding and advertising

♦ Early infiltration and conditioning of sectors of society, e.g., milk given to school-age children

♦ Medical industry funding

♦ Doctors' and health workers' advice – rarely focused on good nutrition

♦ Medical practitioner training, often heavily reactionary, rather than proactive and preventative

♦ Negative stigmas about raw diets, vegetarianism and veganism

♦ Propaganda about protein and need for fish, meat and dairy products

♦ Erroneous governmental food pyramids and recommendations

♦ Social pressures

♦ Eating as a part of social gatherings

♦ Restaurant menus based around standard American/Western diet (SAD), and the scarcity of vegan/vegetarian restaurants

♦ Giving and receiving food as treats, rewards or love

♦ Eating to please others, your partner or a parent cooking for you, for example

♦ Eating around work schedules, whether you're hungry or not

♦ Stigma about using the bathroom frequently and the belief that eating lots of fruit and vegetables will cause frequent bowel movements

♦ Peer pressure

♦ Lack of time to research into health and good diet

♦ Cancer industry propaganda, which promotes the idea that people are just 'struck down' with cancer rather than seeing a distinctive cause and effect from diet and lifestyle

- ◆ Ingredients in foods that cause overeating, cravings and addictions

- ◆ Appealing food packaging, price and convenience

- ◆ Lack of money, marketing and promotion of fruits and vegetables (when was the last time you saw a TV commercial for bananas?)

- ◆ Lack of availability of fresh, healthy food.

- ◆ Conventional stereotypes and beliefs, e.g., eating meat is manly, vegetarian men are wimps, milk builds strong teeth and bones.

All of the above factors combine to perpetuate a widely held notion about diet and health that suppresses the truth about what humans need to survive, and should be eating to thrive. At every juncture, we are subtly and not so subtly exposed to conditioning that has negative and confusing influences on the way we eat, and often forms our views on health.

Compounding this, there are very few positive influences in our lives to encourage us to eat healthily, in moderation and in a way that supports us in thriving with vital energy.

In order to receive positive health messages in our lives, we have to be proactive. We are not conditioned by society for health, so we have to seek to influence ourselves by reading and researching and being willing to go against the societal norms. You can also seek out a coach to help and support you in this area. I know you're willing to do this since you're reading this book, so that's great news.

I recently went to the wonderful and first-ever Thai Fruit Festival, organized by my friend and health activist Harley Johnstone (known as Durianrider). I spent two weeks with around 250 other people, all of whom are thriving on a healthy plant-based diet. Instead of getting drunk and eating junk food, we spent two weeks eating fruit at park gatherings and cycling up mountains. It was a great experience.

❧ Alkaline-delicious tip ❧

Surrounding yourself with a peer group that holds you to a higher standard and supports your healthy lifestyle will work wonders in helping you stay on track.

❧❧

The importance of living alkaline foods

An abundance of living alkaline foods (mainly raw vegetables and fruits) is in harmony with the body's needs. As I described in Chapter 1, alkaline foods help to maintain our blood at a slightly alkaline pH 7.365, whereas eating acidic foods causes a low-level emergency internally because it forces the body to make withdrawals of alkaline minerals from other places (such as bones) in order to maintain correct pH.[1]

So it's not surprising that eating lots of alkaline living foods results in great energy, health and vitality, because you are giving your body what it needs, whereas acidic foods work against your body and make you feel tired, lethargic and unhealthy.

The phrase 'you are what you eat' was derived from Anthelme Brillat-Savarin in 1826 when he wrote, in Physiologie du Gout, ou Meditations de Gastronomie Transcendante, 'Tell me what you eat and I will tell you what you are.' Later, in 1863, in an essay titled Concerning Spiritualism and Materialism, Ludwig Andreas

Feuerbach wrote: 'A man is what he eats.' The actual phrase emerged in English some time later in the 1920s and 30s, when the nutritionist Victor Lindlahr, who was a strong believer in the idea that food controls health, said, 'Ninety per cent of the diseases known to man are caused by cheap foodstuffs. You are what you eat.'[2] In 1942, Lindlahr published the book *You Are What You Eat: How to Win and Keep Health With Diet.*

What Brillat-Savarin, Feuerbach and Lindlahr were telling us was that the food we eat has a great bearing on our state of mind and health because the food we eat goes directly into creating new physical cells in our body. In other words, the food you put inside your mouth and ingest, makes up your hair, nails, organs, muscle, brains, skin, teeth, etc., and directly affects your energy, mood, powers of concentration, weight, health, ability to cope with stresses, speed of ageing and happiness or lack of it.

Think about it: the food we eat goes directly into creating new physical cells in our body.... So, having just given this proper thought, do you really think that eating a piece of chocolate cake, or reconstituted and processed chicken nuggets, or GMO soya, or refined hydrogenated vegetable oil could possibly create healthy new cells or cleanse and nourish existing ones?

Would you fill a fish tank with sewage water? Of course not. You'd use fresh, clean water. Would you put lemonade in your car's fuel tank? No. So why do we, whilst knowing that our bodies thrive on fresh, living foods, recklessly put all sorts of junk into ourselves and expect to keep our good health?

Eating fresh, unprocessed, living alkaline food is the master key to good health because that is what we are *designed* to run on, as humans. It's our high-octane fuel.

Applying the principle of living alkaline foods

We can best apply the principle of living alkaline foods by focusing on eating lots of organic, fresh, ripe vegetables and fruits as the most dominant foods in our diet (these foods are living alkaline foods).

In addition, your dietary choices should be as natural and simple as possible. Any processing, cooking, pickling, freezing, microwaving or refining decreases or completely denatures the nutrients in your food.[3] The exception to this is juicing and making smoothies from fruits and vegetables because, whilst this is refining to some extent, the nutrients are retained and actually more easily absorbed by the body.

❧ Alkaline-delicious tip ❧

Fruits and vegetables are mostly carbohydrates (along with essential vitamins, minerals and water), which means you'll also be keeping your fat and protein intake pretty low in ratio on the A5D.

❧❧

Therefore, I recommend eating a high-carbohydrate, low-fat, low-protein, plant-based diet. This echoes the diet protocols of Dr Douglas Graham's ground-breaking book *The 80/10/10 Diet*, which is based on calories and eating 80 per cent of your calories from carbohydrates, 10 per cent from fats and 10 per cent from proteins. Dr Doug Graham is an expert in natural hygiene and the raw alkaline lifestyle, and he created the 80/10/10 principle for optimum health. I would recommend reading his book for his in-depth look at how to eat a 100 per cent living raw diet.[4]

However, I appreciate that this suggestion may pose some immediate questions or aversions for you, as it does for most people. Having had the privileged insight into people's views on the alkaline diet and how easy or difficult they perceive it to be over the past seven years, I have seen pretty much every question and excuse under the sun as to why following an alkaline diet is too scary or difficult or boring or weird, despite their sincere wish to be healthier and more vital. I should also note that many people's initial aversions are quickly replaced with excitement, enthusiasm and persistence, once they see how simple this lifestyle is and how quickly the benefits are reaped.

Later in this chapter, I'll dispel the common myths and give my top tips and advice for how to live the alkaline diet lifestyle easily, consistently and with success. First, however, let's look at how we can eat for optimum health every day. Simplicity is the ultimate sophistication, so we're going to keep things very simple. That way, you're much more likely to adopt these practices into your daily routine over the long term.

These eating suggestions are simple but require diligence and some discipline to start with, so you may want to work up to them, if that is best for you. Or you may wish to go straight in and eat in this optimal way straight off – use the approach that works best for you.

The eight recommendations for daily eating

1. Eat 15 portions (or 10–20) raw fruits and vegetables per day

For example: 1 raw carrot, 3 raw florets of broccoli, 7cm (3in) slice of cucumber, 4 cherry tomatoes, 1 stick of celery, 1 glass of wheatgrass juice powder with water (or fresh wheatgrass juice shot, if you grow it), 1 banana, 1 apple, 1 pear, a handful of grapes, 1 orange, 10 dates, 1 grapefruit and 2 other fruits (e.g., mango, half a melon, pomegranate, persimmon, handful of goji berries, kiwi, handful of cherries, handful of strawberries).

There are around 1,250 calories in the above, which is approximately half of the daily calorie intake for males and around two-third for females. Your remaining calories can be taken via other cooked or raw foods of your choice. However, if you're very active, as I am, then you'll need to eat many more calories. For example, I eat around 2,200–2,800 calories per day to maintain my weight.

2. Eat fruit for breakfast

Eat either a selection of fruits or a mono-meal of fruits (e.g., 6 bananas or 20 dates or 2 mangos or 8 oranges) as your first daily meal. Aim for around 600–800 calories.

3. Drink a high-chlorophyll green juice every day

Choose a wheatgrass juice or a leafy green vegetable and fruit juice. This provides the blood with a high amount of plant chlorophyll, which cleanses and rebuilds the blood and cells.[4]

4. Drink at least 2 litres (3½ pints) of pure water every day

I advise drinking only fresh, pure water and herbal teas, but if you need a reminder of how much water to drink, see page 72.

5. Eliminate (or greatly minimize) refined oils from your diet

Refined oils are *any* oils that come in a bottle, including so-called 'healthy' or 'good' oils, such as olive, flaxseed or other cold-pressed oils. Only 10 per cent of your calories each day should come from fats – that equates to around

200 calories (22g/¾oz) and 250 calories (28g/1oz) respectively for women and men. You can obtain this amount even on a diet exclusively of plant foods, with no refined oils whatsoever.

By eating fruits, vegetables, grains and small amounts of seeds and nuts you will obtain all the fats you need, so it is not necessary to eat any refined oils whatsoever. You can easily cook your foods by boiling, baking, steaming or 'frying' in water or in a non-stick pan, so cooking without oil is not an issue, as you'll see in the recipes and meal plans in Part III.

6. Combine your foods properly

To ensure good digestion and absorption of vitamins and minerals from your food, eat fruits alone (on an empty stomach). Eat all the most easily digestible foods first (simple carbohydrates – e.g., potatoes, rice or pasta) before eating the harder-to-digest foods last (proteins, especially animal proteins, if you eat them).

🌿 Alkaline-delicious tip 🌿

Proper food combining will prevent you from feeling bloated, gassy and sluggish, aid digestion and help you lose weight.

🌿🌿

Do not drink any liquids with your meals – even water, as this dilutes your digestive enzymes and inhibits the process. Drink water before your meal or an hour after.

7. Eliminate or greatly limit meat, dairy, fish and processed foods

The Alkaline 5 Diet does not include any meat, fish, dairy, eggs (or any other animal product) or processed food products, but if you can't go without those foods then limit them to less than 20 per cent of your calorie intake (around 200–250 calories per day) and only buy organic varieties. This may be a good way for you to transition into the A5D for a couple of months.

You could try eliminating meat altogether for a month, but continuing with fish. The following month, you could try eliminating fish as well, but continuing with dairy. The following month you could then also eliminate dairy to be fully vegan, which I'd highly recommend.

8. Limit cooked foods

If you want to eat cooked foods, then limit them to potatoes, baked, steamed, stir-fried, stewed vegetables and fruits, soups (preferably home-made), rice, buckwheat, bulgur wheat, millet, pasta, couscous, pulses, cereals and pasteurized and pure fruit juices.

A typical day's food

Here are three examples of a typical day's food for me (the number of portions of fruit and veg are in brackets):

Example 1

Breakfast: Fresh lemon juice in warm water (1 portion); 8 large Medjool dates (1 portion); 1 pomegranate with grated apple, lime juice and cinnamon (3 portions)

Calories: 700

Lunch: 2 bananas (1 portion); 6 dates; freshly cut vegetables – broccoli, carrot, cucumber, red pepper, celery (5 portions); 400g (14oz) of boiled potatoes or home-made baked oven chips (fries)

Calories: 950

Dinner: Grapefruit (1 portion); big green salad with fresh mango and tomato dressing (2 portions); wheatgrass juice in 500ml (18fl oz) of water (1 portion)

Calories: 450 calories

Total calories: 2,100

Portions of fruit and veg: 14

Example 2

Breakfast: Fresh lemon juice in warm water (1 portion); large bowl of fresh home-made tomato, aubergine (eggplant) and onion soup (2 portions); 4-banana and kale smoothie (1 portion)

Calories: 600

Lunch: 8 large Medjool dates (1 portion); freshly cut vegetables – broccoli, carrot, cucumber, red pepper, celery (5 portions); green smoothie (2 portions)

Calories: 850

Dinner: 1 apple, 1 pear, 500g (1lb 2oz) grapes, 1 mango (4 portions); wheatgrass juice in 500ml (18fl oz) of water (1 portion)

Calories: 650 calories

Total calories: 2,100

Portions of fruit and veg: 17

Example 3

Breakfast: Wheatgrass juice in 500ml (18fl oz) of water (1 portion); medium bowl of oat and fruit muesli with coconut or almond milk; 2 bananas (1 portion)

Calories: 650

Lunch: 10 large Medjool dates (1 portion); big green salad with spinach, lettuce, tomatoes, cucumber, red pepper, celery (5 portions) with hummus; 1 apple (1 portion)

Calories: 900

Dinner: 1 litre (1¾ pints) green juice from kale, spinach, cucumber, celery, parsley, lime and apples (4 portions); 4 rye crackers with watercress, tomato, ½ avocado and sweet chilli sauce (3 portions); 2 large Medjool dates (1 portion)

Calories: 650

Total calories: 2,200

Portions of fruit and veg: 17

Calories and eating enough

I tend to eat 2,200 to 2,800 calories per day, depending on how much exercise I do. I burn an average of 800 calories at the gym or running on most days, so adjust my calorie intake accordingly. For example, if I want to lose weight I might eat 2,400 calories and burn 800 calories. Or to maintain, I would eat 2,600 calories and burn 500 calories.

One of the easiest ways to modify your calorie intake is with dates and bananas. If you need to eat an extra few hundred calories, add 5 large Medjool dates or 3 bananas. In the Alkaline 5 Diet there is a daily meal consisting of dates and bananas for fat loss and enhanced performance (see page 176).

It is also a good idea to monitor your daily calorie intake and expenditure when you start out, as one of the biggest challenges when changing your diet to one made up of mostly fruit and veg is simply eating enough. You'll find that the sheer volume of food you need to eat to reach your required daily calorie needs is much greater. It is a common mistake for people on a raw food diet to *think* that they are eating lots, but when they add up the calories, it can actually be fewer than 1,500 or 1,000 a day and, as a consequence, they feel tired and disillusioned that they are not reaping the high energy rewards promised.

For example, in a burger and chips (fries) meal, there are roughly 1,000 calories. You'd have to eat 10 bananas, 25 whole lettuces or 25 large Medjool dates to match that in calories.

Be aware of the common stigma of eating too much, as other people may see you eating several bananas and say you're being greedy. However, it seems that our perceptions about foods – mainly from advertising – are a little confused. For example, may people think it's perfectly normal to eat a family-size bag of crisps (chips) or a 200g (7oz) bar of chocolate, but eating 4 apples is classed as being greedy, overindulgent or reserved for someone with a huge appetite.

❧ Alkaline-delicious tip ❧

Being aware of other people's skewed perceptions about food will help you overcome the possible negative effect on your mindset. My advice is just to observe them, be amused by them, dismiss them and then carry on with what you're doing.

Common questions and dispelling myths

Q: Aren't carbs bad for you?

A. No, this is a fallacy. Low-carb diets tend to be high in fat and/ or high in protein, both of which are harsh on your digestive system due to the slow transit of food (food hanging around in the gut and colon, which can cause constipation), putrefaction and fermentation. As a result, low-carb diets are not best for achieving optimum health. We are designed to eat carbs – simple sugars are used directly to produce ATP (see page 59), which we utilize as energy.

Q. I have a sweet tooth – I love chocolate and crave sweet things, how do I give this up?

A. We are designed to have a sweet tooth, which can be satiated by eating lots of fruit sugars – dates, bananas, apples, etc. Eat enough fruit and you won't crave the high-sugar-and-fat hit of chocolate. You can combat cravings for refined sugar and high-fat junk foods, such as chocolate, cakes, ice cream and so on by using the following five-fruit solution:

When you feel a craving for something naughty, eat 5 pieces/ portions of fruit and then if you still want the food, eat it. I pretty much guarantee that after you've eaten 5 fruits, you'll no longer want the original naughty food you were craving. So, for example, you could eat 2 bananas, a handful of dates, an apple, a pear, or 3 mangos if you really wanted, or 5 oranges juiced.

Most of the time when we crave sugary foods, it's because we are not eating enough carbohydrates. Eating just one piece of fruit (averaging 100 calories) won't cut it, so we tend to go for dense, high-calorie processed foods instead. By eating 5 portions of fruit (around 500 calories), you'll get a natural, healthy, high-sugar hit.

Q. Aren't lemons acidic?

A. No, they are acidic in physical form, but when metabolized by the body produce an alkaline mineral ash residue, which alkalizes the blood. The same applies to limes and grapefruits.

Q. Where do I get my protein?

A. There is more than enough protein in leafy green vegetables and fruits – remember, only 10 per cent of calories (around 200–250) per day need to come from protein. Plant protein tends to contain complete protein amino acids (protein-building blocks) and is much more easily assimilated by the body, so this is really not a legitimate worry at all. In fact, the real concern should be eating too MUCH protein, which is a very real health issue in the West, as too much can damage your liver and kidneys.

I have been eating a low-protein diet for years and have good, strong muscles – despite being a long-distance runner (which can sometimes cause muscle atrophy) and not particularly diligent with a weights programme at the gym. If you need more convincing – check out the vegan bodybuilding websites. The best source of protein our bodies can utilize is from plant sources, plus they are not highly acidifying, unlike meat protein.[5]

Q. Won't I feel hungry or deprived?

A. No. The key is eating a larger amount of food. There are far fewer calories per gram in fruits and veg than in most other foods, because of their high water content. Therefore you need much bigger amounts. For example, it may seem excessive to a raw food novice to eat 5 bananas, but this is a moderate calorific intake of 500 calories – the same as a large cookie or chocolate bar or burger.

In fact, my mother used to laugh at me setting off to work in the mornings with a whole sack of food for the day – around 5kg (11lbs) of fruit and veg and smoothies. She'd ask, 'How do you eat all that food and still lose weight?'

The answer, of course, is that the food is low calorie and high quality, so it is hard not to lose weight, if that's your goal.

Q. Isn't it best to have warming cooked food in the winter?

A. Not necessarily. Cooked food can be devoid of many of its nutrients (as much as 80 per cent of the vitamins, minerals and enzymes may be lost) and actually causes a low-level immune response because the food's molecular structure has been altered into something that is not easily recognized and assimilated by the body. Cooked plant foods are very rarely better than raw plant foods, but cooked plant foods are always better than raw or cooked animal products and processed foods. Even in wintertime, it is important to eat some living raw alkaline foods every day.

Q. I am dieting, so won't eating high carbs make me fat?

A. Absolutely not. Eating high carb, low fat is the best way to lose weight or maintain a slender body. Fruit sugar is not the same as refined sugar in, say chocolate, ice cream or cakes, but unfortunately gets lumped in the same no-no category for dieters. Plus, the fattening ingredients in the latter are actually the saturated and unsaturated fats.

Fruits sugars are unrefined, combined with lots of nutrients, fibre and water and are good for you. Cake, ice cream, chocolate, etc., are processed products with minimal nutritional value and are highly acidic. Do not make the mistake of thinking fruits are in the same category as these fattening junk foods.

Eating lots of fruit on your low-fat diet will foster a lean and healthy body.

Superfoods and supplements

Many raw food experts promote eating so-called superfoods and using supplements. Camu camu, bee pollen, ormus gold, chaga mushrooms, moringa, bear's claw herb and other weird and wonderfully named things have some purportedly excellent benefits and nutritional qualities, but they are often very expensive. You could be forgiven for thinking that many of these foods are promoted because there is a high profit margin for those people selling them and being affiliated with manufacturers of them, compared to little or no margin in promoting whole fruits and veg.

In my recipes, I occasionally use some superfoods, such as maca or acai berry powder; these add good flavour and are cheaper and easier to find than many others. Generally, the use of these in the recipes is optional and not necessary.

As long as you are eating lots of fresh, ripe, raw, organic, high-quality fruits and vegetables, you will receive all the nutrients that your body needs to thrive. After all, our ancestors did not, and our close relatives the chimps do not have access to superfoods, so it is unlikely that these hard-to-obtain and concentrated foods are essential for us.

However, I would recommend including the following foods in your diet:

- Wheatgrass

- Sprouts

- Probiotics

Wheatgrass

I recommend drinking wheatgrass juice daily because it is packed full of green chlorophyll, which is very similar to our blood's haemoglobin and is a fantastic blood cleanser and cell builder. It contains nearly the full spectrum of nutrients, vitamins and minerals that we need – all in one small potent shot of the juiced grass.

Ann Wigmore famously used wheatgrass extensively in her institute in California to treat terminally ill patients, with much success. She wrote a number of books on the subject, including the excellent *Be Your Own Doctor*. In fact wheatgrass juice has been widely labelled 'nature's greatest healer'.[6]

You can grow and juice wheatgrass yourself, or buy it in powder form and mix with water. Both are inexpensive and in my experience, a great daily investment and insurance policy for your health, vibrancy and wellbeing.

Sprouting

Sprouting beans and seeds, such as alfalfa, broccoli seeds, mung beans, brown (wholegrain) rice, quinoa and bean sprouts, is a good way to get high-nutrient dense plant protein. You can easily spout seeds and beans at home yourself in a few days, or you can buy packs of fresh sprouts inexpensively from health food shops. Sprouts are a good addition to salads, or great eaten on their own as a snack.

Bacterial Balance

The bacteria in the colon, often referred to as 'intestinal flora', is a combination and balance of 'good' and 'bad' bacteria. Any time that you have less than two bowel movements per day, you know that you need to increase your levels of probiotic good bacteria. This can be achieved by adding cultured and fermented foods such as Kombucha tea (which is a great alternative to wine or alcohol) or sauerkraut (which you can make at home from cabbage) to your diet, in moderation, along with high-fibre fruits and vegetables. Avoiding processed and refined fat and sugar foods is the optimum way to maintain a healthy colon.

The benefits of applying this principle

Here are some of the main benefits of eating living alkaline foods:

♦ Feeling alive and vital

♦ Having sustained energy throughout the day

♦ Sleeping well

♦ Weight loss or regulation

♦ Better skin, hair and nails

♦ Bright eyes

♦ Feeling calmer and more able to cope with life's stresses

♦ Properly balanced hunger mechanism and less likelihood of overeating or emotional eating

♦ Being able to eat large amounts of food and not put on weight

♦ Your palate will adjust to living alkaline foods and your sense of taste will become much more sensitive and attuned to the subtle and delicate flavours of a plant-based diet

♦ Refined fats, meat, dairy and processed foods will start to become unappealing or even repulsive to you – making it easy to eat healthily

♦ Greater ability to concentrate and focus

♦ A leaner waist, as less cortisol is produced (and likewise other stress hormones that contribute to abdominal fat retention)

♦ Greater athletic and strength performance

♦ Feeling happier

♦ Looking and feeling younger

♦ Greatly supports the healing process and a healthy immune system

♦ Eating is much easier, simpler and faster because less time and effort is required in preparing and cooking your food

Chapter 8

Ditch the Nasties:
Eliminating Acidic Toxins

The flipside to eating living alkaline foods is eliminating, or at least minimizing, your consumption and use of unhealthy, acidic toxins. These toxins can be classed into two groups:

♦ Food and drinks

♦ Household, beauty and environmental products

It would be a real shame to eat lots of fresh raw fruits and veg and then cancel out their benefits by (sometimes unwittingly) acidifying your body with toxic beauty products, pollutants, foods and drinks. So, here follows a concise list of things you should be mindful of and avoid as far as you can.

The importance of eliminating toxins

There are many things all around us in our daily life that can throw our bodies out of alkaline balance, if we are not aware of them and do not take steps to keep them out of our life as far as we can.

Many of these toxins are heavily marketed by advertisers and some even promoted as being healthy and beneficial. Others are just not labelled as being bad for us. You have to be mindful that there are many people with many different agendas other than health and preventing and curing disease – not least the big pharma companies. This is why we need to be vigilant and take responsibility for our health education.

Acidic toxins directly acidify the body and it takes a lot of 'doing the right thing' to restore your alkalinity. For example, it has been reported that it takes 32 glasses of water to neutralize one can of cola, and it's classed as a highly corrosive substance when in transport.[1]

So it's not quite the case that one 'good' thing balances out one 'bad' thing. You need to be doing a lot more of the right things to ensure a good blood pH is maintained comfortably, without your body having to utilize its 'alkaline buffering' mechanisms to restore homeostasis (i.e. optimum blood pH of 7.365).

Think of it like this: when you are too hot, your body will sweat and your veins will rise to the surface of your skin to cool you down. When you are cold, your body will shiver and get goose bumps in order to get you moving and warm up. This is because optimum body temperature is 37.5°C (99.5°F) and if it deviates from this by only a small amount, you die.

In a similar fashion, when blood pH is constantly erring on the side of over-acidity, your body will be forced to take measures to bring it back to its correct pH. Unfortunately, this means doing things like leeching calcium and other alkaline minerals from your bones and using it to alkalize your blood. If this continues for a sustained period, then diseases like osteoporosis can occur.

It's very clever the way our body does this really – it compromises less vital functions to save the critical ones, and correct blood pH is critical to keeping us alive.

This means that you can go for many years often without having any signs or symptoms of disease or ill-health, but in a low-level state of acidosis. Eventually, your body will not be able to cope any more and this acidosis will manifest into something serious, like an allergy, skin condition, obesity, or one of the big three diseases – cancer, heart disease and diabetes.

Another way for our body to cope with over-acidity in its inner terrain, is by storing excess fat and 'dumping' acidic toxins in there. Often when people follow a more alkaline lifestyle and eliminate toxins, weight loss occurs naturally and pretty effortlessly.[2]

Eliminating acidic toxins, coupled with eating living alkaline foods, is a great health insurance policy. You'll see the benefits almost immediately in terms of vitality and, in the long term, with your longevity.

Applying the principles of eliminating acidic toxins

Here is a concise list of the things that I recommend that you eliminate from, or at least minimize in, your diet and lifestyle:

Food and drink toxins

Caffeine: A neurotoxin and a diuretic.

Soya: It contains phytoestrogens that disrupt hormonal function. Also, unless organic, soya is highly likely to be genetically modified.

Cigarettes: Not a food, but still taken in orally. Obviously, if you are a smoker, giving up is the number one best thing you could do for your health.

Alcohol: Eliminate alcohol from your life or severely limit your intake as it's actually a poison. Many people are amazed how much life improves for the better when they stop drinking. Try alcohol-free beers and wines – they're pretty good.

Sodas: Especially cola drinks which are highly acidic and harmful.

Dairy products: Milk contains many millions of pus cells. The average somatic (pus) cell count in US milk per spoonful is 1,120,000,[3] and, shockingly, has been shown to deplete calcium in our bodies, not replenish it. See the Harvard nurses study of 238,000 nurses for more information on this,[4] or my website article, 'Is Milk Bad For You?' (you'll find the link to this in the Resources section, see page 231).

Meat: The husbandry and slaughter of animals causes them to release a large amount of adrenaline and other stress hormones, all of which makes meat more acidic to our bodies than it already is. There is also the issue of the GMO feed and hormones given to the animals, as well as glues and fillers injected into a lot of processed meat. You can get more than enough and superior-quality protein from plant sources.

Modern factory farming methods used by the meat and dairy industries mean that animals are often kept in pretty bad conditions. This is also the number one cause of our planet's depleting resources and pollution problems. You may want to explore these ethical issues surrounding the consumption of eating meat and dairy to add momentum to you choosing a plant-based diet. This made it a no-brainer for me.

Packaged and microwaved foods: Nutrient-poor, compared to foods in their natural state, and often filled with unnatural preservatives and flavourings.

Cooked foods: Cut down and include a lot more raw living plant foods in your diet. The A5D 21-day meal plan advises eating 20–70 per cent raw foods and the rest cooked foods. So every day you are getting plenty of high-nutrient raw foods.

Fish: Eat sparingly if you are minimizing rather than eliminating and choose wild fish over farmed. High levels of mercury can also be an issue in deep-sea fish, such as tuna and swordfish.

Refined oils and salts: Refining foods makes them too concentrated and therefore not good for us. A diet high in fat can promote and exacerbate diabetes, as it disrupts the blood sugar levels in your cells. You may be shocked to hear this, but diabetes is often a problem of too much fat in a person's diet, not too much sugar. I know many people who have reversed diabetes on a high-fruit (sugar) and low-fat diet. I recommend reading Dr Neal Barnard's *Program for Reversing Diabetes* (see page 231), which covers the subject in detail.

By eliminating packaged and processed foods then you are ensuring that you are not eating all sorts of harmful chemical preservatives, additives, flavours and colourings. Here's a list of some particularly nasty ones to avoid.

♦ Modified maize starch

♦ Aspartame (E951)

- ◆ MSG (E621)

- ◆ Maltodextrin

- ◆ Soya lecithin

- ◆ Sulphur dioxide (E220)

- ◆ Hydrogenated/trans fats, sodium sulphite (E221)

- ◆ High-fructose corn syrup

- ◆ Sodium nitrate and nitrite

- ◆ BHA & BHT (E320)

- ◆ Potassium bromate

- ◆ Food dyes such as E133, E110, E102, E124

This is not an exhaustive list of food additives to eliminate, but suffice to say that you should minimize packaged, processed and refined foods (with the exception of organic vegan packaged goods) because they are a minefield of chemical nasties.

✤ Alkaline-delicious tip ✤

Obviously not all 'bad' foods are equal – it is better to have a home-cooked broth (mildly acidic) than a deep-fried sausage and chips (fries) (highly acidic) and a soda water is better than cola. So be discerning with what foods and drinks you choose if you're not completely eliminating acidic toxins from your foods.

❀❀

Household and beauty products, and environmental toxins

Parabens: Found in a multitude of shampoos and shower products, but you can find many without parabens. Consumer pressure has led many manufacturers to label products that are paraben-free.

Antiperspirants: Contain aluminium, which has been linked to Alzheimer's Disease.[5]

Sodium Lauryl Sulphate (SLS): A surfactant, detergent and emulsifier used in thousands of cosmetic products, as well as in industrial cleaners. It is found in nearly all shampoos, toothpastes, shower and bath products and make-up foundations. SLS been linked to cancer, neurotoxicity, organ toxicity, skin irritation and endocrine disruption.[6]

Microwave ovens: Not only do they denature food, but they harmfully change the food's molecular structure, creating 'radiolytic' compounds and making it potentially carcinogenic.[7] They don't call it 'nuking' for nothing.

Mercury amalgam dental fillings: Mercury is one of the most poisonous substances for us. One of the main dangers is the instability of the mercury in fillings, which can give off harmful vapours. It is a good idea to avoid having any new amalgam fillings, and you may want to consider having your existing ones replaced with white fillings.

Fluoride: Found in most toothpastes, tap water (in some countries, banned in others), canned foods, many beers and wines. Fluoride can damage fertility, destroy bones and cause early puberty in children.[8] Find fluoride-free toothpaste from your local health food shop and filter your tap water, or buy bottled.

Wi-Fi emissions: Electro Magnetic Frequency (EMF) radiation from prolonged Wi-Fi exposure by using your computer, tablet or phone has been shown to cause all types of health problems from impaired concentration and brain function to infertility[9–10] and should be minimized by using an Ethernet connection to your computer for the Internet where you can, instead of wireless. Turn off your wireless router at night as it can disrupt sleep.

❧ Alkaline-delicious tip ❧

Being indoors, in a car or in public transport compromises the quality of your air and limits your vitamin D absorption. Seek to minimize your time indoors and in vehicles by getting outside in the fresh air as much as possible. Cycle or walk as much as you can every day.

The benefits of applying this principle

When you eliminate, or minimize, your consumption and use of toxins, you'll experience the following benefits:

♦   Blood purification

♦   Cleansing of your body both inside and out

♦   A strengthened immune system

♦   Lifted mood and relief from depression

♦   Feeling a zest for life and happy

- Improved liver, gall bladder, kidney and colon function

- Cleared congestion, especially in lungs by reducing mucus

- Better concentration

- Less anxiety and nervousness

- Weight regulation

- Improved skin

- Higher libido and sexual performance

- Delayed signs of ageing – looking and feeling more youthful

- Aids fertility

Chapter 9

Bodies In Motion:
Movement and Posture

We live in a time and society where sitting down at desks and on sofas for long periods of time is a commonplace everyday activity while using cars and other transportation vehicles to get around is the norm.

Our bodies, however, have not evolved for such a sedentary lifestyle. Mechanically, we are designed to be standing, moving, active beings and if we don't pay heed to this we pay the price with our health.

For people who have physically active occupations, such as gardeners, builders, carpenters, sportspeople, customer service staff, cycle couriers, full-time parents etc., keeping actively moving is not an issue, but keeping correct posture could be. For office workers and drivers, both movement and posture can definitely be an issue and, as with your diet, sleep and other aspects of the Framework for Optimum Health and Healing, you need to be mindful and vigilant of your posture, getting your body moving throughout each day.

🦋 Alkaline-delicious tip 🦋

I define movement as anything from walking and cycling to gardening and dancing, but it must be for sustained periods throughout each day.

🦋🦋🦋

Good posture is about your body being 'centred', poised and in correct spinal alignment when standing and sitting so that your spine is upright and your chest open.

The importance of movement and posture

Active movement and correct posture keep your body in good working order and help to maintain the health of your heart and cardiovascular system, lymph system, bones, joints and muscles, your brain, digestive and immune systems.

Good posture is vital in keeping your spine aligned correctly, preventing back pain and ensuring that your nervous system functions well. Bad posture, over time, can result in 'subluxation' or 'pinching' on the nerves by vertebrae that are out of alignment. This can cause a multitude of problems, from headaches and sciatica to mental fog and even depression.

In short, you have to keep your engine ticking over and moving along the right tracks in order to be healthy.

Applying the principles of movement and posture

The easiest way to apply this principle is simply by doing lots of walking every day. I usually walk at least three miles per day, as well as doing harder cardiovascular exercise on top of that.

Walking

Walking really is the perfect exercise: it's low impact, it can be combined with deep breathing and being out in nature, it gets you stood upright, which is great for your posture and, unlike running, does not require a high level of fitness and pretty much anyone can do it.

Get regular walking breaks throughout the day. I usually walk a mile by the sea first thing in the morning, take another mile or so walk at lunchtime and then in the evening I walk some more. In this way, it's not a big, onerous activity and I find it's easier to fit in three 15–20 minute walks a day than one walk of an hour or more. It is also more beneficial physically and mentally to walk little and often than one longer walk because it gives your body a chance to get revved up several times throughout the day and so gets your brain working better too. This really is a great practice for your overall wellbeing.

The very act of standing up and walking means that you have 100 per cent better posture than being sat down. Combine that with walking tall with your shoulders back, chest open and breathing deeply (see page 60), and you'll be doing wonders for your posture too.

Cycling

Like walking, cycling is another fantastic way to get moving: it's low impact, weight bearing and simple. The extra benefit of cycling over walking is that you tend to get more of a cardiovascular workout and burn more calories, so it's a great activity for weight loss. Also, you can cover more distance on a bike, so it can double as a viable alternative to using your car.

Pilates

Great for flexibility and increasing core (abdominal) strength, which helps to improve your posture. Check out the classes at your local gym or have a look online for a simple instructional class that you can do at home.

Good posture in the office

If you're an office worker or spend any amount of time on a computer or sitting down (who doesn't these days?) then make sure that your shoulders are back (expanding your chest) and that your back is straight when you are sitting at your desk. A poor posture collapses your lungs and results in very shallow breathing.

If you are currently using a less-than-optimum chair at your desk, ditch it, bite the bullet and invest in a high-quality ergonomic chair or kneeler to support your spine correctly and keep your posture good. This is one of the greatest investments you'll make – since so many hours are spent at work and your spine and back health is so precious.

If your employer provides your office chair, ask if they can do an ergonomics test for your desk area (this is a legal requirement in many places) to make sure your set-up is safe and healthy.

Even better still, if your workplace allows it, is to work standing up or sitting on a gym ball. Chiropractors and other back and posture experts recommend this. In fact, many experts say that the chair is one of the worst inventions for our bodies in terms of spinal alignment, posture and breathing.

The benefits of applying this principle

Here are just a few of the benefits of getting more exercise and taking care of your posture:

♦ Greater flexibility

♦ Improved cardiovascular fitness

♦ Improved immune function

♦ Anti-ageing

♦ Stronger core muscles

♦ Greater sense of calm and mental clarity

♦ A toned body

♦ Fat loss, when combined with correct diet

♦ Greater connection with nature, which can lead to greater spiritual connectedness

♦ Improved and sustained energy throughout the day

Chapter 10

The Bright Side of Life: Positive Mindset and Emotions

The effect of emotions, feelings, mindset and attitude on your health is tremendous. We all know someone who has a negative attitude and always seems to be bemoaning their lot; their health, energy and demeanour tend to follow suit.

Many diseases are 'psychosomatic' – relating negative mindset and stress with impaired physical wellbeing. Similarly, a positive mindset and attitude relates to positive physical health and being free of disease and illness. At a biochemical level, it has been shown that positive thoughts and feelings are actually alkalizing – they make your body more alkaline, while negative thoughts and feelings cause acidity in the body[1]

It is vitally important that you have a positive mindset, if you want to live the best life that you can; and having a positive mindset is a choice, not an accident. As Abraham Lincoln said, 'We can complain because rose bushes have thorns, or rejoice because thorn bushes have roses.'

The importance of a positive mindset and emotions

A positive mindset means that you have a positive expectation that things will turn out well and that you will succeed. It gives you more courage to try and persist with diet and lifestyle changes than if you have a negative mindset.

Making positive changes in your diet and lifestyle in turn increases your vibrancy, energy and positivity. This strengthened positivity gives you increased courage and persistence to explore other new areas of your life and make other intelligent changes, which in turn can increase your confidence and positivity and desire to stay on a diet that facilitates this positivity – and so the virtuous cycle continues.

❦ Alkaline-delicious tip ❦

In a nutshell, being positive enhances all aspects of your life, which fosters more happiness, and being happy causes your body to become more alkaline.

❦❦

Applying the principles of a positive mindset and emotions

It is almost impossible in our modern age to be 'naturally' positive. There is so much fear, scarcity, violence, resistance, apathy and other negative things thrown at us from every angle – from the television and newspapers to other people who like to commiserate with each other over their grievances. For this reason, it is absolutely necessary to *cultivate* your positive mindset and attitude, which will lead to day-to-day positive emotions.

'How can I do that?' you might be asking. Here's what I've learned over many years from many different seminars, books and mentors, distilled down into one page of guidelines for your convenience and immediate use, on how to live a powerfully positive life.

♦ Start by making the decision that your view of the world is a choice and optimism is a learnable skill. Decide that the world is a positive place and that there is as much good as there is evil. Just decide to release any resistance to this and choose it.

♦ Make a list of 100 things you've experienced in your life that show evidence that the world you live in has many good facets. Acknowledge and decide that your happiness and your fulfilment in life on this earth is *your* responsibility, not that of others. Realize that circumstances do not determine your happiness; it's your *interpretation* of the circumstances and the meaning you attach to them that determines your happiness. As Zig Ziglar said, *'You cannot tailor-make the situations in life, but you can tailor-make the attitudes to fit those situations.'*

♦ Throw away your television. Advertisers and the media are supremely sophisticated in mind conditioning and subliminal messaging techniques, not to mention the plain, pure negativity that is pumped through the news 24/7. From my extensive training in marketing and studying the science of persuasion, I know first-hand just how easy it is to influence human beings to a certain desired action or state of mind. I have watched many sales speakers use systematic, pure science to get people to buy their products – they follow a technique and get the same results every time. Of course, this can be used ethically or unethically, but do you honestly believe that the media, advertisers, politicians and food/medical industries have *your* best interests at heart, when there is so much money, power and control at stake? Do yourself a favour and give yourself lots of extra free time – dump the square box.

♦ Guard your mind and be careful what you allow in. A friend of mine used to say, 'You wouldn't let your neighbour come into your house and dump their rubbish there, so don't let people dump rubbish into your mind,' and this is so true. Our subconscious minds are very powerful and are just that – *sub*conscious. We can't tell the impact something has on our subconscious mind, but we do need to be mindful on a conscious level of what we allow into our mind.

♦ Read uplifting materials (*not* magazines and newspapers), watch uplifting videos (*not* TV), listen to music that is inspiring you (*not* standard pop and rock music). This can really enrich our day-to-day experience of life.

♦ Be proactive, rather than reactive. Other people and circumstances will always demand your time – emails and phone calls to answer, expectations of friends and family, colleagues and clients. Schedule some 'me' time, but also structure your day to get your high-value, high-priority things done and the less important yet 'urgent' tasks done afterwards.

♦ No one will give you permission to live life on your terms; you have to take charge and demand it of yourself and others around you.

◆ Surround yourself with good, kind, supportive, successful, uplifting, positive people. Distance yourself from negative types – the complainers, moaners and naysayers – even if they might have been long-standing friends. Their negative effect on you is much more pervasive than you think.

◆ Talk to yourself positively and guard against speaking negatively to, or about, yourself. Be your own champion. You, more than anyone else in your life, need and deserve that and doing this helps you to be the best you can be for other people too.

◆ Don't gossip or moan about other people. If you have a problem with someone, speak to them directly.

◆ Help others as much as you can and go out of your way to extend compassion. For example, give to charity or tithe, help homeless people and volunteer.

◆ Keep your word and keep agreements as far as you can. This will maintain your esteem both in your eyes and other people's.

◆ Live a balanced life: work hard on what you enjoy doing, spend quality time with friends and family, exercise often, spend time in nature, be fun and silly, enjoy your hobbies, discover/develop your spirituality and faith by joining a prayer or meditation group, for example.

◆ Be grateful – give thanks and praise often and actively think of at least 10 things each day (ideally morning and evening) that you are thankful for in your life and that have happened that day. An attitude of gratitude is a great way to get you instantly onto a positive vibe and to be more resilient to life's everyday stressors.

Having a positive mindset and emotions is not about being happy all the time – allow your emotions to be, whether positive or negative, and let them pass, don't allow yourself to get attached to them. It is rather an overall conviction that whatever happens, I'll handle it.

The benefits of applying this principle

A positive mindset and outlook will improve your life in every way and you will experience some distinct health benefits, including:

♦ Increased longevity

♦ Reduced risk or symptoms of depression

♦ Lower levels of distress and anxiety

♦ Greater resistance to the common cold

♦ Greater immunity in general

♦ Better psychological and physical wellbeing

♦ Reduced risk of cardiovascular disease

♦ Better coping skills during times of stress and hardship

♦ Greater resilience and resourcefulness

♦ Better communication and relationships with others

♦ More happiness, fulfilment and meaning in your life

♦ A greater sense of purpose in life

♦ A greater sense of connectedness to your fellow human beings, and spiritually

Part II
The Principles of the Alkaline 5 Diet

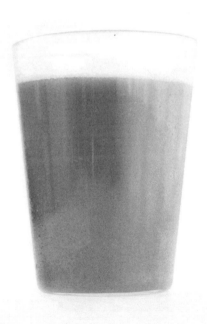

Introduction

Introduction

Get Ready for A5D Success

So, as you have read so far, living a healthy alkaline lifestyle is about much more than just food, but I expect you already knew that. It is about a holistic approach to health and about balance in body, mind and spirit.

Before we move on to the specifics of the Alkaline 5 Diet, I would suggest going back over Chapters 4–10 (see pages 59–126) and making a short action plan, based on each of the elements of the Framework for Optimum Health and Healing:

1. Sunlight and deep oxygenation

2. Pure hydration

3. Sleep and balancing rest

4. Living alkaline foods

5. Eliminating acidic toxins

6. Movement and posture

7. Positive mindset and emotions

For each of these elements, write down two actions that you are going to take in the next week and commit to making them a habit for the next month. This action alone, before getting into the ins and outs of daily meal plans, will invigorate your life greatly. So go and do it now; it is simple and you'll feel good for taking this action.

A5D success stories

To inspire you on your way, here are just a few of the success stories from my website subscribers and people who have tried A5D. These are not uncommon testimonies and I'm sure you'll agree offer many good reasons for trying the diet for 21 days. I have yet to meet anyone who has tried the alkaline diet, or more specifically A5D, and not seen some considerable health and body improvements.

Until about eight years ago I was on a high-protein diet, but not in good health: tired, pale, sickly looking, retaining water and depressed. Then a friend, who owns a health food store, suggested that I check the pH levels of my urine and they were about 4.5 – totally acid. That weekend I went on a broth fast, using vegetables and potatoes and drinking freshly made green juices from my friend's health food store. In two days I lost about 5lbs, the colour began to come back into my skin and I felt like a new person... it was as though a huge weight had been lifted off my shoulders. I began to read books about raw foods and the alkaline lifestyle, and now eat a raw food diet and am careful to monitor my pH level. I use the alkaline diet food list on your website and it has made a huge difference. Since then I have never looked back, but it still amazes me how incredible I feel and how all those crazy and annoying symptoms, like aches, pains, fatigue, bloating, excess weight, have just gone away now that my body is balanced. – ALICIA

I was on high-blood-pressure medication for over 10 years, but have been an alkaline vegan for two years now. During some recent tests, my blood pressure was normal while off medication and, with my doctor's approval, I weaned myself off my meds while monitoring my blood pressure on a daily basis. My blood pressure is now within normal range and I'm off my meds. So much for 'it's in your genes', I am so happy. – GRANT

I've only been using the Alkaline 5 Diet for three weeks, but I truly feel better than ever before in my life. I am convinced of the benefits of this diet and intend to keep on it for life. The weight loss doesn't match anything I have ever, EVER tried before. And believe me, I've done it all! Thank you. – CAROLINE

I did the Alkaline 5 Diet for 21 days and felt amazing. My energy was great and my mind was so clear – I'm a nurse and just felt really on my game. I used an app on my phone to count calories to ensure I was consuming enough. The day I didn't count calories was the only one that my cravings were out of control and I wanted to eat junk foods. I now know exactly how to thrive with my diet and health, and this diet is so simple once you get used to the amount of food you have to eat (which is a bonus!). – GREG

This is ULTIMATE. The HOLY GRAIL of all diets! I am on and off raw (only cooked plant-based dinners), but I still stick to high carbohydrate, low fat, low protein and the results have been phenomenal. We were born with a sweet tooth for a reason – to enjoy an abundance of juicy, sweet, beautiful fruit. Carbs for the win! – ANGELO

I scrupulously followed an alkaline vegan diet for over two years. At 47 years old, it helped me achieve six-pack abs in four months. It is an incredibly high-energy and healthy diet, and extremely easy to do. I stopped for a little while because it made socializing around food nearly impossible. However, for the few months I stopped, I didn't feel as good, gained some fat and lost my abundant energy, so I went back on it. Now I prepare for when I eat out with friends: I eat beforehand and order a salad or a simple rice or pasta or potato dish with fresh vegetables and maybe start with a fruit salad. It's quite easy actually and my friends are all used to it and also getting very interested in my diet. I eat a vegan diet with a tremendous amount of raw fruit and strongly believe the 'fruits and shoots' diet is the natural diet of human beings. If you need to improve your health and looks, this diet will do it in spades. – MARK

The Alkaline 5 Diet worked really well for me in the first three to four months after undergoing a couple of operations for a deadly cancer. All my ailments (I am nearly 60 years old) just melted away: I slept better, lost 36lbs and felt just terrific – and that after a lifetime of horrible ignorant abuse of my body and the highest weight of my life at 16st 12lbs. I researched my particular cancer to learn that only a pH-balanced body can create an environment where these recurring cancer cells (stromal sarcoma-a) cannot survive. I thought I would never be able to maintain eating or living this way, but I was very wrong. I now drink 3 litres of alkalized water per day, have a triple shot of fresh wheatgrass daily, eat an avocado, a lemon, a tomato and as many dark green veggies as I can eat every day. I feel amazing. – PAUL

I've lost 12lbs in two weeks. I know some of that may be water weight, but my clothes feel much looser, my skin looks amazing and I look forward to exercising. I never thought I'd say that! This diet is wonderful because the results are so clear so quickly. My sister-in-law originally told me about it – she has lost over 40lbs in over a year and looks younger than 10 years ago. I am convinced of the alkaline diet and with Laura's five-meal approach, it makes it very simple for anyone to do and stick with it long-term. – CHRIS

I suffered from fibromyalgia; it was very painful and I was almost disabled. Then I read about alkaline water and the body's pH levels. I bought a water ionizer and started drinking about 3 litres (5¼ pints) a day and using it to make herbal tea. Within four weeks, the pain was going away. Within four months I was completely pain-free. I can't make any claim as to whether the alkaline water was responsible or not, but I feel like a new person. – STEPHEN

I had a big open sore in the middle of my tongue for about four years due to suffering with collagenous colitis and could hardly taste any of the food I ate. Since I have been alkalizing, it is disappearing and is only a small mark now. How do I thank you for your wonderful work? Thank you, thank you, thank you! – ANNEKE

I did the Alkaline 5 Diet for 21 days and lost 10lbs in that time. The only hard part for me was the Fat-Loss Sugar Meal because it meant eating tons of bananas and dates, which are very sweet. However, it did stop any cravings, so I see its purpose and my energy levels were very high. Thanks for showing me how to easily attain my goals. A5D is something sustainable that it's possible to do day in and day out for an unlimited number of days, as well as a jumpstart to great health. – KIM

Well – I'm feeling good and have more energy, clearer thinking and a lighter spring in my step. I don't have any scales, but I know I have lost some weight; I can feel it. My day will now always begin with lime or lemon in water and I will be adopting the green juices each day. The bananas and dates are lovely and energy-giving, and my children have got used to seeing 20 or more bananas on the countertop. I am finding more ways to enjoy a plate of vegetables and my soup-making is getting better too. Overall, a great success and my old habits have changed. Thank you, Laura, for being the inspiration and the guide, the example of the possible, the light into my shadows, much appreciated. – ROBIN

I started with predominately alkaline foods to help with a stomach condition and am having good results so far and hoping to do without meds soon. Thankfully I have been largely vegetarian for years now, so don't think there'll be too much of a transition problem… it's really just ingraining it now. I am feeling great at the moment and it's pretty easy! – CATHY

In 2002, I had an accident at work that caused a Chiari Malformation (this is where the cerebral tonsils drop down into your spinal column and prevent spinal fluid from flowing properly into your brain). I had seven surgeries within six months in 2004 to try to correct this and developed hydrocephalus. After the sixth surgery, I developed an MRSA staph infection and this was followed by meningitis. I nearly died. For the next five years, I got debilitating migraines and was in and out of the emergency department every month. Doctors told me that was just how it was going to be and there was nothing more that could be done. I couldn't accept that and started doing my own research into health and nutrition. A friend told me about the alkaline diet when he was diagnosed with inoperable lung cancer. He had been told that there were reports that cancer can't grow in an alkaline body. He tried the diet and became cancer-free. I decided to see if it would help with my health issues too. After a week I was off all my pain meds. I haven't been to the ER in more than a year and am working full-time again. I haven't been on any prescription drugs for more than six months. When my mother saw how my health had turned around, she decided to try it for her health issues – she had debilitating fibromyalgia and was taking drugs, including morphine, up to 10 times a day and was still in pain. After three days on the alkaline diet, she was off her pain meds. I have become a huge supporter of alkaline living and hope that more people give it a try. Thank you for your work and videos, I often click the 'share button' and post to all my friends. I hope more people discover the amazing benefits of the alkaline diet. – SHARI

Chapter 11

The Basics of the Alkaline 5 Diet

A5D is made up of low-fat plant foods only, which are mostly alkaline-forming and work in harmony with your body's pH balance, and so keep us healthy and slim. It is also known as a low-fat (raw) vegan or high-carb (raw) vegan diet because it excludes any meat, fish, dairy, bee products or refined oils – all of which are acidifying because they contain harmful levels of saturated fat, too much protein, cholesterol, infectious organisms or harmful and genetically modified chemicals.

You eat at least one food option from each of the five 'meal' categories every day, as well as drinking at least 2.5 litres (3½ pints) of pure alkaline water each day.

Herbal teas, mineral water, fresh fruit and vegetable juices, coconut water, small amounts of coconut or almond milk are permitted on this diet; all other drinks (including alcohol and caffeine) are not. That said, once or twice per week you could include a Kombucha tea, fruit cordial or non-alcoholic wine or beer – as long as they only contain high-quality natural ingredients.

In terms of calories, aim for 80 per cent calories from carbs, 10 per cent from fats and 10 per cent from protein. This is a well-documented and proven ratio for optimum health, energy and performance, as pioneered by Dr Douglas Graham in his book *The 80/10/10 Diet* (see page 90). The good news is that by eating a fruits-and-vegetables-based diet, you naturally follow the 80/10/10 principle.

Guidelines for success

Raw: 30–80 per cent

This includes a combination of 30–80 per cent (by calories) raw fruits, vegetables and leafy greens, as well as cooked vegetables – such as potatoes and vegetable soups – and whole grains and wholegrain products – such as rice, pasta, couscous and bulgur wheat. In this way, you get the maximum nutrients from the fruits and vegetables *and* the benefits of a raw food vegan diet. The addition of some cooked carbs makes the diet easier to maintain.

Seeds and nuts

You can also include a small amount of soaked nuts and seeds. I'd suggest eating about 50g (1¾oz) or less per week.

Natural condiments

You can use herbs, spices, small amounts of sugar and salt, vinegars, chutneys (relishes), pickles, purees, sauces and other condiments, as long as they are vegan, GMO-free, low fat and free of any additives, flavourings and colourings – 'natural' or otherwise – or anything else with a chemical-sounding name.

Easy-prep fast food

You will need to prepare the vast majority of the food yourself, so that it's 100 per cent natural and there are no 'mystery' ingredients. The good news is this is the ultimate fast-food convenience diet. It's very easy to prepare your meals, eat on the go and clean up afterwards. How hard is it to prepare a mono meal of dates or whiz up a 5-banana smoothie in your blender, for example?

No assumptions

Many people assume that a vegan lifestyle is extreme or will be difficult due to the belief that it will be inconvenient or expensive or that they will feel deprived in some way, without even trying it. Actually a vegan lifestyle is quite the opposite: it is the most satisfying, energizing, abundant and convenient diet there is; you just have to experience it for yourself.

I recently spent two weeks in Thailand with 200 other high-carb vegans and we were all in agreement that this diet and lifestyle is one of ease and abundance. That's not to say that it's always easy to eat out in restaurants and socially – it's not, unless you live in Thailand where vegan restaurants are plentiful. So for this reason, I would say that it's probably best to avoid eating out for at least the initial 21 days on A5D.

> *Thanks to you, Laura, I am just about to hit my two-year alkaline vegan anniversary. I was never a vegetarian, so went straight to vegan for a month's trial. Wow, it's a great lifestyle. You look great and are a great advertisement for the vegan lifestyle. Keep running and singing! –* Robert

You might be concerned about food cravings, but because you will be getting all your nutrient requirements, you will soon find that you are no longer subjected to the powerful addictive elements in so many common foods and won't crave fatty, sugary or processed or refined foods. Many people also find that their monthly food bill goes down, their energy and digestive functioning improves and it's actually easier to follow this diet than having to prepare, cook and clean up after standard Western meals. Try it for at least 10–21 days and then form your opinion, not the other way around.

What's more, there is plenty of evidence to support the fact that we, as human beings, should *only* be eating plants – not only because it's best for the animals and the environment, but best for our health too. There is no propaganda needed to support this viewpoint – unlike the meat and dairy industries that spend billions each year lobbying the health service, pushing their agenda and influencing our food choices, often in a very negative way, towards a diet high in refined and saturated fats.

Finally, if you have any doubts about whether the vegan lifestyle is a healthy one, please watch any of the eye-opening and interesting documentaries listed in the Resources section (see page 231).

The key to health success is in the details

It's the subtle differences that make the big differences in the diet and health game – the biggest and most important game you'll ever play in your life. Lose your health and pretty much everything else goes with it. Maintain your health and you can have a good and active life. Optimize your health and you can live a life of abundance and joy.

Here's what I mean by the subtle differences. Let's use John and Jane as an example.

John and Jane are both having curry and rice for dinner. John's is made with a bottled sauce that contains MSG, (genetically) modified maize starch and 50 per cent of its calories from refined oils. He adds some lean chicken that's been fed a putrid mix of crushed cow bones and GMO corn and serves it with some fried white rice.

Jane's curry is made with freshly steamed vegetables, spices, a little almond milk and a can of chopped tomatoes. She adds some chickpeas and sweet potato and serves it with boiled brown (wholegrain) rice.

The taste and feel of the meal for both is warming, spicy and satisfying, but there's a huge difference between the two curries: John's is highly acidifying and contains many fattening and potentially harmful ingredients, whereas Jane's is healthy, naturally low in fat and energizing.

Or take another example.

John and Jane both fancy a sweet treat. John grabs a bag of toffees and a chocolate bar. Jane grabs two bananas and a pack of dates. They both eat around 700 calories, but John's treat contains GMO soya lecithin, saturated milk fat, flavourings and preservatives, and leaves him feeling sluggish after eating it. Jane's treat is very low fat, high in fibre, 100 per cent raw and natural so it satisfies her sweet cravings, digests very easily and makes her feel great for the rest of the day.

There is a huge difference between, for example, two different bottles of tomato ketchup – one might contain just tomatoes vinegar, salt, sugar and spices while another might contain modified maize starch, flavourings, MSG, etc., and so potentially be damaging to your health.

The message here is to take care with your food choices and read the labels of commercially prepared foods. By choosing natural plant foods, you won't have to do this nearly as much, because fruits and veg don't have labels.

Best for weight loss

Did you know that not all calories are created equal, and that 2,500 calories of natural plant foods and whole grains is not the same as 2,500 calories of burgers, ice cream, chocolate, lasagne and pastries? When you switch getting your calories – from fatty sugary and refined processed foods to plant sources – for a significant amount of time you literally 'turn off' the fat genes in your cells and this will help you lose weight.

Dr Neal Barnard, whom I mentioned earlier (see page 24), is a medical doctor, founder of the Physicians Committee for Responsible Medicine and author of six books, including *Turning Off the Fat Genes.* His work and research has shown that fat genes are highly influenced by our diet, and the types of foods we eat determine how fat or thin we are rather than any genetic or inherited traits:

> *'Everybody has a gene for fat storage, which is located on chromosome 8, and its effects become obvious on our thighs and waistlines. But it essentially shuts off, if you keep fat out of the foods you eat. If your fat-storage machinery has nothing to work with – no fat to store, that is – it quits.... In our research we use low-fat, vegan diets and find that the resulting weight loss is about 1 to 1½ pounds per week, week after week after week. We also see dramatic*

improvements in cholesterol. We reported last year in the American Journal of Cardiology the greatest cholesterol lowering ever found in women under 50.' It occurred in 5 weeks, simply using a low-fat vegan diet.'[1]

A word on fruits and carbohydrates

Avoid getting sucked into all the marketing hype about low-carbohydrate and low-sugar foods being healthy. Simple science refutes this – our cells run on sugar. We need glucose molecules to convert to ATP for energy and you can be fairly certain that obesity clinics and dentists' chairs are not being overburdened by raw vegan fruitarians.[2]

By its nature, eating a low-carb diet means eating foods that are high in fat and/or protein – both of which disrupt our digestive system and put a heavy burden on our organs such as liver, heart and bowels.

If you want great digestion, to lose weight and/or maintain a slim and toned physique, sustained energy throughout the day and good sleep, you must eat a high-carbohydrate diet. More specifically, you must eat a diet with plenty of fruit and vegetables, and some cooked, starch carbs, such as potatoes, rice or pasta.

Fruit sugar and diabetes

Dr Neal Barnard also wrote the ground-breaking book *Program for Reversing Diabetes*, based on the research he and his colleagues conducted over many years – the most notable funded by the National Institutes of Health and published in the August 2006 issue of *Diabetes Care journal*.[3,4] Dr Barnard's programme has been found to be three times *more* effective at controlling blood sugar than the American Diabetes Association dietary guidelines. He recommends eating fruit in abundance – it's the meat and dairy that's the issue. Here's what he says:

'Load up on beans, vegetables, and fruits. Choose whole grains (try barley, oats, quinoa, millet, wholewheat pasta, etc.). Aim for at least 3 grams per serving on labels and at least 10 grams per meal. Choose unlimited amounts of grains, legumes, fruits, and vegetables.'

Chapter 12

The Alkaline 5 Diet Meals

The A5D makes it easy for you to get all your nutrients and none of the harmful acidifying foods, in five memorable steps, with five easy meals.

Each meal type has been optimized nutritionally for good digestion, as well as taste and satiation. You simply pick one option from each of the five meals every day:

1. Blood Cleanser (BC)

2. Vitamin Vitality Meal (VVM): 15 per cent of your daily calories

3. Fat-Loss Sugar Meal (FLSM): 10–70 per cent of calories

4. Raw Alkaline Mineral Meal (RAMM): 5 per cent of calories

5. Hearty Cooked-Fibre Meal (HCFM): 10–70 per cent of calories

As you can see, there is flexibility between the FLSM and the HCFM; a good rule of thumb is to have 50 per cent raw and 50 per cent cooked calories per day – so you'd have 50 per cent calories from HCFM, 30 per cent calories from FLSM and then the given ratios for the others. The Blood Cleanser (BC) contains negligible calories, so counts as zero.

Establishing your daily calorie needs

To work out your specific calorie needs – adjusted very accurately to your age, weight, height, levels of activity and desire to lose, gain or maintain weight – you need to know your current weight in pounds and your height in inches.

1. Work out your basal metabolic rate (BMR)

This is the number of calories you need to maintain your body weight by just the metabolic process, not factoring in any activity you may do.

BMR Formula Women

BMR = 655 + (4.35 × weight in pounds) + (4.7 × height in inches) – (4.7 × age in years)

BMR Formula Men

BMR = 66 + (6.23 × weight in pounds) + (12.7 × height in inches) – (6.8 × age in years)

2. Determine your total daily calorie needs

To calculate this, multiply your BMR by the most appropriate Harris Benedict Formula[1] number, as follows:

♦ If you are sedentary (little or no exercise): Calorie-Calculation = BMR × 1.2

♦ If you are lightly active (light exercise/sports 1–3 days/week): Calorie-Calculation = BMR × 1.375

♦ If you are moderately active (moderate exercise/sports 3–5 days/week): Calorie-Calculation = BMR × 1.55

♦ If you are very active (hard exercise/sports 6–7 days a week): Calorie-Calculation = BMR × 1.725

♦ If you are extraordinarily active (very hard exercise/sports and a physical job or 2× training): Calorie-Calculation = BMR × 1.9

3. Calculate calories required to lose or gain weight

To work out the calorie consumption you need to lose or gain weight, take the number you calculated using step 2 (your calorie needs for weight maintenance) and adjust as follows:

♦ For weight loss – subtract 500 calories per day from this number.*

♦ For weight gain – add 500 calories per day to this number.

♦ For weight maintenance – do nothing and use the number from step 2.

Write down your target daily calorie intake.

*The American College of Sports Medicine (ACSM) recommends that calorie levels should never drop below 1,200 calories per day for women or 1,800 calories per day for men. Even these calorie levels are quite low.[2]

There are approximately 3,500 calories in a pound of stored body fat. So if you create a 3,500-calorie deficit through diet, exercise or a combination of both, you will lose one pound of body weight. If you create a 7,000-calorie deficit you will lose two pounds and so on. The calorie deficit can be achieved either by calorie-restriction alone, or by a combination of fewer calories in (diet) and more calories out (exercise). This combination of diet and exercise is best for lasting weight loss. Indeed, sustained weight loss is difficult or impossible without increased regular exercise.

Your five daily meals on A5D

Drink the Blood Cleanser first thing, on an empty stomach. You can then eat the other meals in any order you prefer, but it is important to remember the following two rules:

◆ Drink 500ml (1 pint) of pure water before each meal (except the Blood Cleanser – drink 500ml/1 pint of water 20 minutes afterwards).

◆ Eat fruit on an empty stomach (at least 2 hours after the previous meal) and on its own or before your Raw Alkaline Mineral Meal or Hearty Cooked-Fibre Meal.

Here follow the details about each of the five daily meals.

1. Blood Cleanser (BC)

Drinking a highly alkalizing blood cleanser is the best way to start your day. This will give you a double whammy of benefits: cleansing your blood and liver while providing lots of nutrients and giving you energy for the day ahead.

Wheatgrass juice (powdered or fresh)

Wheatgrass juice is a fantastic blood cleanser and builder because it contains green plant chlorophyll, which is only one molecule different to our blood's haemoglobin and harnesses sunlight energy. Wheatgrass is known as nature's panacea and was used by Dr Ann Wigmore extensively in her Natural Health

Institute for detox and healing. You can read more about the benefits of wheatgrass and where to buy it by checking the Resources section (see page 231).

Green vegetable juice

You can juice any leafy greens or other green veg you like, such as lettuce, spinach, kale, cucumber, celery, cabbage and Brussels sprouts. High in green plant chlorophyll and sunlight energy, green juices provide a great start to the day.

Lemon juice in warm water

This is a great liver and urinary tract cleanser too and highly alkalizing (remember, it's the mineral ash that's left behind in your body that makes a food acidic or alkaline; lemons leave an alkaline ash). Simply juice one whole lemon and add 200ml (7fl oz) of warm water. Don't use boiling water or it will denature the nutrients and enzymes. Drink for a refreshing morning zing that freshens your breath, regulates your appetite and gives a good dose of vitamin C first thing.

2. Vitamin Vitality Meal (VVM): 15 per cent of calorie allowance

You can think of this meal as your vitamin pills and supplements delivered in a flavourful, complete, pretty package, just as nature intended – called fruits. Quite simply we are designed to eat large amounts of sweet fruits every day. Our body is set up for it, in terms of our digestive system and physical make-up, and is the reason for the tongue's sugar receptors. In nature, we would easily and naturally be able to find, 'catch' and eat a fruit, unlike eating an animal.

There are various ways to eat your fruit – whole or as a fresh juice or smoothie. To really get the most out of your fruit you will need a blender and a juicer, as both are essential equipment for any health enthusiast to have in their kitchen. However, if you don't already own these items then consider buying an inexpensive blender to start and then, as you carry on longer-term, upgrading to a high-speed blender and a 'masticating' juicer, which squeezes rather than spins the fruit to obtain juice.

Fresh Fruit

A VVM meal could consist of a mono-meal of six oranges or five pears, five apples or 450g (1lb) of grapes, or a mix of a few different fruits.

Eat your fruit when it's fully ripe and buy organic whenever possible, so that you get the maximum nutrients and taste from it without any potentially harmful chemicals.

Fresh fruit juice

Freshly squeezed or juiced at home is the best juice to drink. Second to that, freshly squeezed or pasteurized shop-bought juice is acceptable, and good as a backup when you get caught out feeling hungry or can't find a better alternative. Go for fruit juice and carb yourself up rather than being tempted to reach for something not within the parameters of this optimum diet lifestyle. Remember, we're aiming for 80 per cent of calories from carbs, 10 per cent from fats and 10 per cent from protein.

Simply throw your favourite fruits into a juicer – you can go for a single fruit juice, such as orange or pineapple, or mix a few fruits together. As a general rule don't mix citrus fruits (e.g., oranges, lemons and limes) with sub-acid fruits (e.g., apples, grapes or cherries). Also, melons should be juiced on their own. As long as your fruits are organic or washed well, you can leave the skins on them – even pineapples, lemons and oranges, but not mangoes.

🌿 Alkaline-delicious tip 🌿

Pasteurized juice is cooked, so if you're looking to follow a high-raw version of A5D then strictly it should not be included in your Vitamin Vitality Meal. Check the labels of any commercially bought juices and avoid any that include the words 'from concentrate', as they lack both the fibre and nutrients of 'fresh juice'.

Fresh fruit smoothies

I prefer fruit smoothies to juices because there is less waste and you retain all of the fibre, which also helps fill you up. Simply blend a mix of your favourite fruits together for 30 seconds. Try a blend of 2 bananas with a large handful of blueberries, a pear and an apple. Experiment and then enjoy all the fruity goodness.

Green smoothies

A delicious blend of fruits and some leafy green vegetables can be a great alternative to all-fruit juices and smoothies because it provides minerals, protein and calcium from the raw greens while still tasting sweet and fruity. Experiment with different blends. One of my favourites is a blend of 3 apples, a handful of spinach leaves and a head of lettuce.

Dried fruit with NO additives or preservatives

It can be difficult to find quality dried fruit (except perhaps for dates) that is 100 per cent fruit, with no additives or preservatives (e.g., sulphur dioxide, a type of sulphite that can cause or irritate asthma and allergies[3]) in mainstream supermarkets and grocery stores. However, if you can find unadulterated dried fruit, it's fine to include in this meal. You can generally find high-quality dried fruit online and it makes it cheaper to buy in bulk too.

Coconut water

Coconut water – fresh from a coconut or shop-purchased – is a mildly sweet, fresh-tasting, healthy drink and can make a great addition to your banana smoothies. Make sure it's 100 per cent coconut water and nothing else. This is not the same as coconut cream or milk, although you might want to include some coconut milk as a milk substitute on this diet.

Stewed fruit

Stewed or pureed fruit can also make a warming meal. Fruit compotes or jams made with only fruit and fruit juice are also useful additions. Steer clear of jams and fruit prepared with added refined sugar and pectin. They are a backup plan or 'treat' only.

3. Fat-Loss Sugar Meal (FLSM): 10–70 per cent of calorie allowance

A banana and dates meal should be a staple in your diet every day, unless you live somewhere like Thailand where you can get an abundance of tropical fruits easily and all year round, in which case you could replace this meal with other fruits.

The reason that this meal is included is that it is very hard to get enough calories on a vegan diet, in particular carbohydrate calories, without eating a lot of nuts and seeds or other oils (which are not high carb). Therefore, fruit is the perfect food because it provides plenty of vitamins, water and sugar that we can use as our fuel for energy.

Bananas and dates are delicious when they are fully ripe, but, more importantly, are sweeter and denser in calories than most other fruits. For example, you'd have to eat 12 oranges to get the same calorie content as a 6-banana smoothie, which contains about 600 calories.

Many fruits are full of water and the number one mistake that many people make when following a low-fat vegan diet is not eating enough. If you don't eat enough calories, then you are liable to fail because getting too hungry leads to making unsuitable food choices and grabbing the nearest thing to hand. Eating bananas and dates keeps you walking the right path and it is my number-one strategy for dealing with hunger or craving.

♦ If I fancy a chocolate bar, I eat bananas or dates.

♦ If I fancy some alcohol, I eat bananas or dates.

♦ If I fancy a cake, I eat bananas or dates.

♦ If I fancy bread, I eat bananas or dates.

♦ If I fancy a pizza, I eat bananas or dates (or my Hearty Cooked-Fibre Meal, see page 158).

♦ If I fancy some nuts, I eat bananas or dates.

♦ If I fancy something fatty, I eat bananas or dates.

♦ If I fancy some ice cream, I eat frozen banana 'nice cream' (see recipe on page 202).

The craving for the original food goes every time (which suggests the need for carbohydrates) and has the added bonus of not creating any of those sluggish and bloated feelings afterwards, unlike the original fattening, unhealthy choice. What's more, the FLSM is designed to help you put an end to any 'emotional eating', cravings and overeating, and maintain steady energy levels.

Getting your food ratios right

Your FLSM meal should make up 10–70 per cent of your calories and your Hearty Cooked-Fibre Meal (HCFM) should make up the other 10–70 per cent. So, the total for both should equal 80 per cent of your daily calories. Here follow some examples of the ratio of FLSM to HCFM:

♦ 50 per cent dates: 30 per cent rice meal.

♦ 30 per cent bananas: 50 per cent potatoes.

♦ 40 per cent bananas and dates: 40 per cent rice meal.

Some examples for a 2,000-calorie intake day might be:

♦ 1,250 calories dates: 750 calories rice meal.

♦ 750 calories bananas: 1,250 calories potatoes.

♦ 1,000 calories bananas: 1,000 calories rice meal.

When you first start the diet, aim to eat 50 per cent of your daily calories from raw foods. That means that the ratios for your FLSM and HCFM should be 3:5–30 per cent FLSM to 50 per cent HCFM, which is a good ratio to start with. The 21-day A5D meal plan in Part III is in line with these ratios. If you want to maximize the nutritional benefits, simply increase your raw intake as you become more accustomed to the diet, after the 21 days.

What if I don't want to lose fat?

If you have no extra weight that you want to lose, that's fine. Maybe you're very lean already – an athlete or bodybuilder or have always been slender. If this is the case, the FLSM becomes your High Performance Sugar Meal. As well as aiding fat loss – due to curbing cravings and being low fat and tasty – bananas and dates are also a premium food for both mental and physical performance and recovery, due to their high nutritional value.

Your High Performance Sugar Meal is simply the FLSM with more calories – you can add extra bananas and dates to this meal and you can also add more to your Hearty Cooked-Fibre Meal.

Bananas

Simple, convenient, delicious, super-healthy and relatively inexpensive, try to buy organic when you can and eat them only when they are ripe – brown and spotty. This is when the full range of vitamins, minerals and sugar has had time to develop, as well as when bananas are at their lovely, best flavour.

Some people might worry that they are eating too much potassium by eating lots of bananas, but this really is not the case. You'd need to eat and digest around 100 bananas in a minute to overload your body with this mineral. Many long-term banana fruitarians have had their blood tested and their potassium levels are just fine. Potassium is also great for anti-ageing.[4]

Dates

As well as sugar, dates contain an optimum amount of protein, fats, vitamins A and B, minerals such as iron, magnesium and potassium. They are classed by many experts as a perfect food and used by people across the world to break fasts[5] because they are easy to digest and contain simple sugars, which satiate hunger quickly, as well as delivering lots of vitamins and minerals. Be mindful that they must be 100 per cent dates with no preservatives.

My favourites dates are Medjool, Deri and Deglet Noor and you can buy them in bulk online and in most major supermarkets and grocery stores.

You'll find lots of banana and date recipes and ideas for your Fat-Loss Sugar Meal in the 21-day meal plan (see pages 173–226).

4. Raw Alkaline Mineral Meal (RAMM): 5 per cent of calorie allowance

This meal delivers a full spectrum of amino acids, which are much more easily assimilated by the body than animal proteins, vitamins and minerals, and are a better source of calcium than dairy.[6] Leaving the vegetables raw means they retain all of their nutrients and enzymes. Buy organic when you can and make sure you wash the vegetables thoroughly before cooking.

❧ Alkaline-delicious tip ❧

Think of this meal as your health insurance policy and beauty regime all rolled into one, as eating plenty of raw vegetables will give you clear skin and bright eyes, and so help keep you looking and feeling youthful inside and out.

A big green salad is a wonderful addition to your daily diet, especially if you want something salty. It always surprises me just how much I enjoy munching on a green salad once I get into it. You can make a low-fat salad dressing with various condiments such as mustard, agave syrup, apple cider or balsamic vinegar, herbs and spices, lemon or lime juice.

🌿 Alkaline-delicious tip 🌿

Eating plenty of raw veg will keep your digestive system running smoothly and, given you're doing so much to improve your health, also gives you a little leeway to have the occasional naughty (vegan) treat, such as a few squares of dark chocolate or a fresh bread roll and jam.

Green Vegetable Juice

I am not particularly fond of green veg juice, except for wheatgrass juice, which I love. However, I do like the energy kick I get an hour or so after drinking it. It's an instant and very alkalizing nutrient boost. A green juice is also a beautifying drink. The chlorophyll and minerals have anti-ageing properties and can give your skin and eyes a real glow, not to mention healthy-looking hair.

I like to juice my leftovers when I have cabbage, sprouts, kale, spring onions (scallions), beetroot greens, celery, cucumber or spinach that need to be used up. Add enough vegetables to make about 200ml (7fl oz) of juice. This is a relatively small amount, but keep in mind that this juice is packed full of nutrients and is very potent.

5. Hearty Cooked-Fibre Meal (HCFM): 10–70 per cent of calorie allowance

This meal will be your secret weapon, as it will help you to keep on track and eating a low-fat, alkaline, plant-based diet long after the 21 days. I know this to be true because for years I wanted to eat 100 per cent raw vegan, but found myself craving cooked food. I am happy to eat just fruits and veg in warmer climates, but I live in the UK where it's colder and I find it more difficult to stick to 100 per cent raw food.

However, I made the mistake of thinking that I had to eat raw vegan 100 per cent or nothing. In other words, if I couldn't stick to raw plants then I might as well just fall off the wagon and eat anything – dairy, chocolate, pizza, etc.

This is a classic mistake we make: aiming for gold standard (raw fruits and veg) and feeling like a failure when we don't quite make it, and so giving up. However, the silver is still up for grabs and within our reach, and this is where the HCFM comes in. I've been eating this way for years now and I love this meal because it's just so satisfying and simple.

The HCFM is also a great digestive tract and colon cleanser. If you're used to eating meat and dairy then you'll immediately notice an improvement in your bowels as your movements will become more frequent and your stools will be softer and easier to pass.

✿ Alkaline-delicious tip ✿

When you start eating a low-fat vegan diet, you quickly find that your tastes change. You begin to appreciate simple, subtler-tasting dishes, which are made from only a few ingredients, rather than the taste-overloaded processed foods with their artificial, overpowering and addictive flavourings and additives. So try this way of eating for 21 days, or 10 days at the very least – with no expectations or pressure on yourself to continue after 21 days. Remember, no assumptions!

☙❧

Cooked starches with a flavourful sauce

The principle of the HCFM is to have a satisfying cooked starch with a low-fat sauce or dressing made of only natural ingredients. To add great flavour, you can use herbs, spices, curry powder, small amounts of sugar and salt, vinegars, chutneys (relishes), pickles, purees, sauces and other condiments. The only thing to remember is that they should be:

♦   GMO-free

♦   Low fat

♦   Free from additives, colourings, flavourings (including 'natural' flavouring)

♦   Vegan

♦   Organic, if possible

I prefer to keep it very simple by just having, say, some boiled couscous or brown (wholegrain) rice with a few vegetables, some mango chutney (relish) or sweet chilli sauce or an organic vegetable stock cube and spices. Warming, satisfying and very tasty. The key is to experiment with different sauces. To start, you may prefer a stronger-tasting sauce, but it's likely you'll soon start to appreciate a simpler, subtler flavour.

Make HCFM a luxurious ritual

You can make your HCFM a more luxurious ritual by serving your food in attractive bowls – mine are small and ornate, so that I can have second and third helpings and feel very indulgent. This is similar to the traditional Asian way of eating (and, as we know from The China Study,[6] their diet is great, see page 24).

Put on some relaxing music – I'd suggest classical as it has a proven calming frequency[7] – and really enjoy your meal by eating slowly and tasting every mouthful. Eating this way makes mealtimes more indulgent and satisfying, plus it aids digestion and nutrient absorption.

I like to have my HCFM for breakfast and find it a great way to start the day. For 20 or more years, I ate on the go, rushing, whilst watching TV, etc. It's only recently that I have learned to sit and enjoy my food, and feel grateful for it and its nourishment. I am a slow learner on this front.

Here is the selection of cooked starches that you can choose from for this meal.

Potatoes or sweet potatoes

Baked, steamed, boiled or added to vegetable soups, potatoes are very versatile and satisfying. You can even make your own oven-baked potato wedges, which are as delicious as a bowl of chips (fries), but are low-fat, gluten-free, cheap, a vegetable source of fibre and starch and contain the correct amount of plant protein and fats (see recipe on page 193). If you buy commercially available oven chips (fries), just make sure that the ingredients are just potatoes and a *little* vegetable oil, nothing else.

Rice

Organic brown (wholegrain) rice is best and makes a simple, delicious and inexpensive meal. I like to have a big bowl of brown (wholegrain) rice with veg and spices or with a little rice wine vinegar, organic brown (wholegrain) rice miso and organic sweet chilli sauce with a leaf of wakame (seaweed) for breakfast – yum!

Pasta

Most people love a pasta dish and you can eat it guilt-free on A5D. Wholegrain organic pasta is best. It's also inexpensive, and quick to cook. Teamed with a tasty tomato or pepper-based (bell pepper) sauce, it makes a delicious meal.

Quinoa, couscous, millet, buckwheat and bulgur wheat

Any dishes you would make with pasta, potatoes or rice, you can also substitute quinoa, couscous, millet, buckwheat or bulgur wheat instead. They are all low-fat, complex carbohydrates and have the optimum proportion of protein and essential fats – around 10 per cent of both in each.

I like to switch between these grains for a bit of variety in the week. Also, some grains take more time to cook than others – for example brown (wholegrain) rice takes around 30 minutes to cook, but couscous only takes a few minutes. So if I want my meal sooner, I'll choose couscous.

Vegetable soup or stew

Vegetable soups and stews are tasty and filling, but bear in mind that vegetables are much lower in calories than grains, so you have to eat much more to get your desired intake of carbohydrates and nutrients. To get 600 calories from a vegetable soup, you will need to eat about three large bowls, compared to one medium-sized bowl of rice.

If you prefer, you can always add rice or pasta to your vegetable soups to make a risotto-style or casserole dish.

Wholegrain crackers

Make sure your crackers have just a few simple and natural ingredients – such as rye and salt. Team them with a home-made avocado and tomato guacamole or salsa (see recipe on page 193) or chickpea hummus. These dips are all fairly low fat since you're not adding any oil, but don't have more than 2 to 3 avocados per week as they are quite high in calories.

🌿 Alkaline-delicious tip 🌿

If you can find a good local wholemeal (wholegrain) organic bread (made with flour, water, salt and yeast) or make your own bread, then this is OK to include in your HCFM. Commercial breads with a longer shelf life tend to have all sorts of additives and preservatives in them, as well as milk derivatives and lots of salt. For this reason, I'd advise keeping bread to a minimum. Root vegetables and grains are a far more nutritious way to eat your cooked starches.

Pulses

You can add lentils, beans, peas and chickpeas to your HCFM, but they shouldn't be the main bulk of your meal because they are higher in fat and protein (usually only around 68 per cent carbs). Make potatoes, rice, pasta, quinoa, millet or couscous the main portion and add around 30g (1oz) of pulses for a bit more body and variety in taste and texture.

100 per cent raw or more cooked food?

The beauty of this diet is that it caters for your needs whether it's for a short 100 per cent raw vegan cleanse (for example a seven-day, fruit-and-veg-juice-only cleanse), or if you're dedicated to eating 100 per cent raw all the time. If you are facing a severe health challenge then personally, I would start doing this immediately.

To do this, simply replace your Hearty Cooked-Fibre Meal with another Fat-Loss Sugar Meal or Vitamin Vitality Meal. Since cooking food causes it to lose as much as 80 per cent of its nutrients, going 100 per cent raw offers superior nutritional intake from your food.

Conversely, if you want to add more cooked food to the A5D then you can. I don't necessarily recommend it, but some people may prefer to make a transitional stage from the standard Western diet.

In this case, simply replace half of your calories from your Fat-Loss Sugar Meal with another Hearty Cooked-Fibre Meal. So, for example, if your average daily calories from your FLSM are 1,000 calories, eat 500 calories as your FLSM and have the other 500 calories as a second HCFM.

Tips to help you on your way

Split up meals

You do not have to eat all of your allocated calories for each meal in one go. For example, your HCFM is generally 50 per cent of your daily calories. For a fairly inactive woman, this would equal 1,000 calories. Eating 200g (7oz) of cooked grains with some vegetables, spices and a dollop of chutney (relish) would be around 1,000 calories, but you might choose to eat half of this meal in the morning and half later in the day.

The same goes for the other meals too, as you can spread them throughout the day. This might mean having three small FLSMs. Just make sure that you follow the food combining rules and eat fruit on its own.

Combat the cold

If you feel the cold or live in the cooler northern hemisphere, then eating more raw food is likely to make you feel colder. This is a common issue and certainly true for me. Overcome the cold by wearing layers of clothes and make yourself a hot water bottle to cuddle up with in the evenings. Once you know and prepare for this, it's easy to stay warm and cosy.

Urinary and bowel movements

Drinking lots of water and eating water-rich fruits and veg means that you will be urinating often. It may seem like an inconvenience, but is a sign of good health. You should be urinating at least 10 times per day and it should be light straw- or clear-coloured – not yellow. You should be having two to four bowel movements a day.

Be prepared for other people

Be aware that most people will think that your new diet and lifestyle is a little strange and will not, necessarily, agree with what you are doing. On top of that, they may give you their well-meaning, albeit misinformed, opinions about not getting enough protein or calcium by following this diet. All of a sudden, everyone becomes a diet expert when you say you're on a vegan diet.

To be fair, veganism is not the mainstream way of thinking or practice. So you may need to develop a certain level of resilience and anticipation when it comes to what others will think of this and the questions they might ask you – as much out of their curiosity as anything. Or you may wish to keep it to yourself, especially when you're just starting out.

When you make a change, it throws up all kinds of issues for friends and family. Especially if that change highlights some things that deep down they know they should probably be doing too, or at least considering.

For example, unless your friends and family are particularly well-educated or enlightened about nutrition and diet, it is natural for them to try to persuade you to go back to what you were doing before – to keep being part of the 'pack', so that they don't feel like you've changed and are leaving them behind. Respond with compassion to other people and be open in your responses to them, rather than defensive.

Use a calorie counter

You can calculate your daily calories and nutrients using a free online tool such as www.cronometer.com. This will help you keep on track of the calories you are eating and make sure your ratios of carbohydrates to fat and protein are 80:10:10.

Take vitamin B12

The only nutrient that is scarce on the A5D diet – and indeed *any* diet, both vegetarian and omnivorous – is vitamin B12 (also called cobalamin), which is needed for good brain and nervous-system functionality. A deficiency can lead to things like pernicious anaemia. We cannot manufacture it in the body and only bacteria can make it.

In the fullness of time, you may want to consider getting your B12 levels tested to ensure you don't have a deficiency, and I recommend taking a supplement – either a sublingual spray or tablet, or an injection. Although, if you eat a lot of organic produce, you may find that you are getting sufficient B12 because it is found in rich soil, so you may be getting traces this way.

Catch some rays

Make sure you get out in the sunshine and fresh air for a walk at least once a day. Keep your arms and/or legs uncovered for about 20 minutes then you can absorb the sunlight energy and produce the amount of Vitamin D you need. If you plan staying in the fresh air longer than this, then make sure you cover up or apply a natural sunscreen after 20 minutes to avoid sunburn. In the wintertime, you may need to eat more foods rich in vitamin D such as mushrooms or take a good-quality supplement.

Beyond the 21 days

After you have completed the 21-day diet and truly experienced the low-fat vegan lifestyle of the Alkaline 5 Diet, you may wish to adopt it full-time. I would certainly advocate this 100 per cent. It is a totally sustainable diet, as well as being great for your health, great for the planet and great for the animals too. You will also continue to experience new benefits long into the future, as so many people do.

If you do decide to adopt this lifestyle, it's a great idea to find your local vegan group or meet-up – or start one yourself. This will help you feel part of a community of like-minded people and it is a fantastic way to make new friends and share meals and ideas.

In the past there has been somewhat of a stigma attached to being vegan. Vegans were portrayed as being hippies who listened to folk music, had long underarm hair and wore tie-dyed clothes. This is a pretty outdated stereotype, and if you adopt the vegan lifestyle you'll be in the company of numerous A-list celebrities: Brad Pitt, Natalie Portman, Jared Leto, Mike Tyson, Pamela Anderson, Casey Affleck, Alicia Silverstone, Garth Brooks, Ted Danson, Ellen DeGeneres, Demi Moore, Jason Mraz and Joaquin Phoenix, to name but a few, all follow a vegan diet and look great on it.

The tide is now changing; there is a rise in this way of thinking and living and you can be the next shining, vital, healthy, beautiful example.

Portion size

The 21-day A5D meal plan is based around eating 2,000 calories per day and will likely result in significant weight loss, whether you exercise or not. If you are a large man and/or do a lot of physical work then please adjust the portion sizes upwards by 500 to 1,500 calories per day (see page 146 to calculate your daily calorie needs).

Do not go below the recommended portion sizes or you will burn out and not succeed with the 21 days or beyond. Rest assured, if it's your aim to lose weight then you will do so by eating abundantly, without feeling hungry or as if you're restricting yourself. In fact, what other diet do you know where you can eat such generous portions of food and lose fat while improving your health and wellbeing all at the same time?

Stocking up your food cupboards

Starches

Here's a basic shopping list of some of the foods you'll need:

♦ Brown (wholegrain) rice

♦ Buckwheat

♦ Bulgur wheat

♦ Couscous

♦ Millet

♦ Porridge oats

♦ Quinoa

♦ White and sweet potatoes

♦ Wholegrain noodles (egg-free)

♦ Wholegrain rye crackers

♦ Wholegrain spaghetti/pasta

♦ Wholegrain spelt spaghetti

Seasonings

- Agave syrup
- Balsamic vinegar
- Basil
- Black pepper
- Brown sugar (organic, unrefined)
- Cider vinegar
- Cinnamon powder
- Coconut sugar
- Cumin powder
- Fresh root ginger
- Ground ginger

- Mango chutney (relish) plus other chutneys (relishes)
- Oregano
- Sea salt
- Tamari soy sauce (organic)
- Thai sweet chilli sauce
- Tomato ketchup
- Tomato purée
- Turmeric powder
- Vegetable stock cubes
- Wholegrain mustard

Fresh fruit and veg

- Apples
- Apricots
- Aubergines (eggplant)
- Avocados
- Bananas
- Basil leaves
- Beetroot

- Blueberries
- Broccoli
- Brussels sprouts
- Butternut squash
- Cabbage
- Carrots
- Cauliflower

- Celery
- Cherries
- Coriander (cilantro) leaves
- Courgettes (zucchini)
- Cranberries
- Cucumber
- Garlic
- Grapefruit
- Grapes (white and black)
- Green beans
- Kale
- Leeks
- Lemons
- Limes
- Mangoes
- Medjool, Deri and Deglet Noor dates
- Melon (all varieties)
- Mixed salad leaves
- Mushrooms
- Olives
- Oranges
- Pears
- Peppers (bell peppers)
- Pineapple
- Pomegranates
- Raspberries
- Red and white onions
- Red chard
- Spinach
- Spring onions (scallions)
- Strawberries
- Sweetcorn
- Tomatoes
- Watercress

Basically any of your favourite fruit and veg, preferably organic and whatever is in season, if possible.

Drinks

♦ Almond milk

♦ Coconut milk (carton, not concentrated in a can)

♦ Coconut water

♦ Fresh vegetable and fruit juices

♦ Herbal teas

♦ Kombucha tea

♦ Wheatgrass powder or juice

What to expect on the 21-day diet

You are just 21 short days away from making some lifelong positive changes to your diet, nutrition and overall health. The first week of the diet, and certainly the first few days, will be about getting used to the recipes and the volume of food you need to eat, and observing how your body and mind feels.

I've included some recipes to get you started; *each makes one serving* unless otherwise stated.

If you prefer to use cup measures rather than metric or imperial, use an online site to quickly and easily convert your measures.

Part III
The 21-day Alkaline 5 Diet Programme

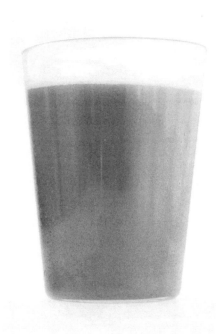

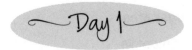

Day 1

1. Blood Cleanser

Juice one whole lemon and add to 200ml (7fl oz) of warm water.

2. Vitamin Vitality Meal

1 litre (1¾ pints) freshly squeezed orange juice. If you want to make this yourself rather than buying it, you'll need around 15 oranges to produce a litre (1¾ pints) of juice.

Calories: 500

3. Raw Alkaline Mineral Meal

You'll be surprised how you'll come to love eating raw vegetables. I take a bag of crudités with me every day to work or to have as a snack after the gym or a run. Simply eat five of your favourite fresh-cut raw vegetables or pick five veg from the following list:

   3 florets of broccoli

   3 florets of cauliflower

   2 carrots, sliced into batons

   5 cherry tomatoes

   1 stick celery, sliced into batons

   5cm (2in) stick of cucumber, sliced into batons

   ⅓ red, green, orange or yellow pepper (bell pepper), deseeded and sliced

Calories: 150

4. Fat-Loss Sugar Meal

Banana Green Smoothie

Adding greens to your smoothies really boosts their nutritional quality and you won't even taste them. This is my standard post-run recovery meal; it helps my muscles to recover quickly and reduces aching – especially if I've done a particularly long or hard run. I think this is the ultimate sports drink, and a much healthier alternative to commercial sports drinks and protein shakes that are often full of additives and preservatives.

> 5 ripe bananas, peeled
>
> 100ml (3½fl oz) water or coconut water (optional, for a thinner consistency)
>
> Handful of fresh kale or spinach
>
> 1 large or 2 small dates, pitted (optional, for extra sweetness)

Place the bananas, coconut water (or milk), kale and dates in a blender and blitz for 30 seconds. Pour into a glass and enjoy its goodness. For maximum nutritional value, it is best to prepare your smoothies when you are about to drink them, rather than make them for later, as this prevents oxidation and loss of nutrients.

Calories: 500 (600 with dates and coconut water)

5. Hearty Cooked-Fibre Meal

Vegetable Cumin Brown (wholegrain) Rice

This is a lovely warming rice dish that's perfect to eat anytime and very easy to prepare. High in taste and nutrients, it will satiate your hunger and give you lots of energy. Use any vegetables that you prefer and preferably ones that are in season.

   150g (5½oz) brown (wholegrain) rice (uncooked weight)

   3 large mushrooms, sliced

   1 stick celery, finely sliced

   5cm (2in) courgette (zucchini), finely sliced or cubed

   3 broccoli florets, chopped

   ¼ red pepper (bell pepper), deseeded and finely sliced

For the sauce

   1 vegetable stock cube, crumbled

   ½ tsp turmeric powder

   ½ tsp cumin powder

   ½ tsp cinnamon powder

   1 tbsp agave syrup

   ½ tsp black pepper

Place the brown (wholegrain) rice in a saucepan, cover with boiling water then cook according to the packet instructions (usually around 30 minutes). In the last 5 minutes of cooking, add the mushrooms, celery, courgette (zucchini), broccoli and red pepper (bell pepper). To make the sauce, place the stock cube, cumin, turmeric, cinnamon, agave syrup and black pepper in a bowl and stir until thoroughly combined. Drain the rice and vegetables before returning to the heat and gently stirring in the sauce until it is well combined. Serve immediately.

Calories: 700

✖ Alkaline-delicious tip ✖

Most major supermarkets, grocery stores and health food shops stock an excellent range of organic whole grains, but you might find it cheaper to buy them in bulk online; it also saves you having to carry lots of grocery bags home or to your car.

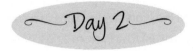

Day 2

1. Blood Cleanser

Juice one whole lemon and add to 200ml (7fl oz) of warm water.

2. Vitamin Vitality Meal

2 apples

2 oranges

1 pear

Calories: 300

3. Raw Alkaline Mineral Meal

Activator Green Smoothie or Ginger Activator
Green Smoothie

This delicious blend of fruits and vegetables is my standard go-to green smoothie. After drinking it, you'll find that you enjoy a real boost, both mentally and physically.

2½cm (1in) slice of pineapple

2 apples, peeled and cored

5cm (2in) slice of cucumber

½ stick celery

Large handful of spinach or kale

Juice of 1 lime

½ avocado (optional), pitted

150ml (5fl oz) water, or more if you prefer a thinner consistency

2½cm (1in) piece of fresh root ginger, peeled (optional)

Roughly chop all the ingredients, place in a blender and blend for 1 minute. If you want to add more zing to your smoothie then include some fresh ginger, I call this 'Ginger Activator Green Smoothie' and it is quite delicious

Calories: 400 (300 without the avocado)

4. Fat-Loss Sugar Meal

200g (7oz) Medjool dates

1 ripe banana

Calories: 700

5. Hearty Cooked-Fibre Meal

Bulgur Wheat Cabbage Wraps

Bulgur wheat takes much less time to cook than brown (wholegrain) rice and gives you variety in your grains. It is inexpensive and widely available from major supermarkets, grocery stores, health food shops and online. These cabbage wraps are delightfully tasty as the crunchiness of the cabbage goes well with the chewy nuttiness of the bulgur. Plus you'll be getting an extra hit of raw green veg, which is always a bonus.

150g (5½oz) whole or cracked bulgur wheat (uncooked weight)

3 large mushrooms, finely diced

1 stick celery, sliced

¼ red pepper (bell pepper), deseeded and finely sliced

2.5cm (1in) slice of aubergine (eggplant), finely diced

3 large outer leaves of Savoy cabbage

For the sauce

- 1 vegetable stock cube, crumbled
- ½ tsp turmeric powder
- ½ tsp cumin powder
- ½ tsp cinnamon powder
- ½ tsp black pepper
- 1 tbsp agave syrup

Place the bulgur wheat in a saucepan, cover with boiling water then cook according to the packet instructions. In the last 5 minutes of cooking, add the mushrooms, celery, red pepper (bell pepper) and aubergine (eggplant). To make the sauce, place the vegetable stock cube, turmeric, cinnamon, black pepper and agave syrup in a bowl and mix thoroughly. Drain the bulgur wheat and vegetables and return to the heat. Add the sauce, stirring well until evenly mixed. Divide the mixture between the Savoy cabbage leaves, and roll up each wrap. Serve immediately.

Calories: 700

🌿 Alkaline-delicious tip 🌿

It is quite normal to experience some detox symptoms in the first few days. You will be eating a very clean diet and your body will take the opportunity to 'clean house' and expel toxins from your system. So, you may get a few headaches, skin breakouts and tired spells; they are a small short-term tribulation that will yield to amazing long-term benefits, so don't sweat it.

🌿🌿

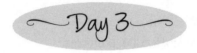

1. Blood Cleanser

Juice one whole lemon and add to 200ml (7fl oz) of warm water.

2. Vitamin Vitality Meal

   2 apples

   2 oranges

Calories: 250

3. Raw Alkaline Mineral Meal

Activator Green Smoothie (see recipe on Day 2, page 179)

Calories: 400 (300 without the avocado)

4. Fat-Loss Sugar Meal

   200g (7oz) dates

Calories: 600

5. Hearty Cooked-Fibre Meal

Vegetable Spaghetti Marinara

This is a super-easy, throw-together and very tasty alternative to the classic Italian dish and without the meat and cheese, you'll feel satisfied after eating without feeling stodgy and sluggish. It's full of herby tomato flavour, with a sweet edge.

   150g (5½oz) wholegrain or spelt pasta or spaghetti
   (uncooked weight)

2 tomatoes, finely chopped

4 mushrooms, finely chopped

½ stick celery, finely chopped

5cm (2in) slice of courgette (zucchini), finely chopped

⅓ red pepper (bell pepper), deseeded and finely chopped

For the sauce

2 tbsp tomato purée

1 tbsp agave syrup

Pinch of mixed Italian herbs

Pinch of sea salt and black pepper

Place the spaghetti in a large saucepan and cover with boiling water then cook according to the packet instructions. In the last 5 minutes of cooking, add the tomatoes, mushrooms, celery, courgette (zucchini) and pepper (bell pepper) to the pan. To make the sauce, mix together the tomato purée, agave syrup and mixed Italian herbs and then season to taste with salt and pepper. Drain the pasta and vegetables well, return to the heat and pour over the sauce. Gently toss the pasta and vegetables in the sauce for about 1 minute, or until well combined. Serve immediately.

Calories: 700

✨ Alkaline-delicious tip ✨

Since rice, potatoes and the other cooked carbs in A5D are generally inexpensive, indulge your taste buds by buying a selection of fine organic chutneys (relishes) from local farmers' markets. Although be careful to read the labels before you buy because more of the smaller producers are now using modified maize starch.

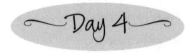

1. Blood Cleanser

Juice one whole lemon and add to 200ml (7fl oz) of warm water.

2. Vitamin Vitality Meal

1 ripe medium pineapple, peeled, cored and chopped into chunks

Calories: 450

3. Raw Alkaline Mineral Meal

Fruity Green Salad with Apple and Avocado Dressing

The addition of cranberries gives this tasty green salad an added twist, and the apple and avocado dressing gives it a lovely creamy texture and flavour.

     2 large handfuls of salad leaves

     5cm (2in) cucumber, finely sliced or diced

     5cm (2in) celery, finely sliced or diced

     Handful of cranberries

For the dressing

     ½ medium avocado, peeled and pitted

     2 handfuls of spinach

     ½ apple, peeled

     Pinch of cayenne pepper

     300ml (10fl oz) water

     Pinch of sea salt and pepper

Place the salad leaves, cucumber, celery and cranberries in a large bowl and combine gently. To make the dressing, place the avocado, spinach, cayenne pepper and water in a blender and blitz for 1 to 2 minutes. Season the dressing with sea salt and freshly ground black pepper to taste before pouring it over the salad. Toss the salad gently in the dressing until all the vegetables and berries are coated. Serve immediately.

Calories: 300

4. Fat-Loss Sugar Meal

Banana Blueberry Smoothie

The addition of blueberries to your banana smoothie makes a delicious FLSM drink with a juicy tang.

> 5 ripe medium bananas
>
> 200g (7oz) blueberries

Place the banana and blueberries in a blender and blitz for 30 seconds. Serve in a smoothie glass and drink immediately.

Calories: 550

5. Hearty Cooked-Fibre Meal

Vegetable Cumin Brown (wholegrain) Rice (see recipe on Day 1, page 176)

Calories: 700

❧ Alkaline-delicious tip ❧

Keep going with your first week. The overall attitude to adopt for this week is one of curiosity, so go with the flow, be open to the new experiences and changes you're making to your diet, and be interested in how this differs from how you're used to eating and feeling.

❧❧

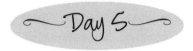

Day 5

1. Blood Cleanser

Juice one whole lemon and add to 200ml (7fl oz) of warm water.

2. Vitamin Vitality Meal

1 litre (1¾ pints) of freshly squeezed orange juice. If you want to make this yourself rather than buying it, you'll need around 15 oranges to produce a litre (1¾ pints) of juice.

Calories: 500

3. Raw Alkaline Mineral Meal

Big Green Sweet Mustard Salad

This salad is easy, tasty and has a clean, sweet dressing that is full of flavour and will really satiate your appetite.

    2 large handfuls of spinach leaves

    1 large beef tomato or 5 cherry tomatoes, sliced or diced

    5cm (2in) cucumber, finely sliced or diced

    ¼ red pepper (bell pepper), deseeded and finely sliced

For the dressing

    1 tbsp apple cider vinegar

    1 tbsp wholegrain mustard

    1 tbsp agave syrup

Place the spinach leaves, tomato, cucumber and red pepper (bell pepper) in a large bowl and gently combine. To make the dressing, mix together the apple cider vinegar, wholegrain mustard and agave syrup. Drizzle the dressing over the salad and toss gently to combine. Serve immediately.

Calories: 300

4. Fat-Loss Sugar Meal

5 medium bananas

Calories: 500

5. Hearty Cooked-Fibre Meal

Vegetable Bulgur Wheat and Mango Chutney (Relish)

Having a good selection of chutneys (relishes) is one of my secret weapons on A5D, as they really add a burst of flavour and variety to your HCFM. Choose varieties with only natural ingredients (no GMO, flavourings or additives).

150g (5½oz) whole or cracked bulgur wheat (uncooked weight)

3 large mushrooms, finely diced

1 stick celery, finely diced

5cm (2in) courgette (zucchini), finely diced

3 broccoli florets, finely chopped

2 medium tomatoes, finely chopped

For the sauce

1 vegetable stock cube, crumbled

1 tsp cumin powder

2 tbsp mango chutney (relish) or sweet chilli sauce

½ tsp cinnamon powder

½ tsp black pepper

1 tbsp agave syrup

Place the bulgur wheat in a saucepan, cover with boiling water then cook according to the packet instructions. In the last 5 minutes of cooking, add the mushrooms, celery, courgette (zucchini), broccoli and tomatoes. To make the sauce, place the cumin, mango chutney (relish), cinnamon, black pepper and agave syrup into a bowl and mix thoroughly. Drain the bulgur wheat and vegetables, return to the heat then stir in the sauce until it's well combined. Serve immediately.

Calories: 700

🌿 Alkaline-delicious tip 🌿

Don't expect to be perfect – it's likely that you'll end up under-eating or not quite getting your calories right – but don't worry, as it is all part of the process and is like learning any new skill; which is what A5D is all about – learning the new skill of eating for optimum health and effortless fat loss. This is a skill that you can reap the benefits of for life. Remember, if you find that you can't eat your HCFM all in one sitting, feel free to split it into two smaller portions and eat one later in the day. If you get hungry then add more bananas or dates to your daily diet.

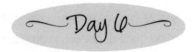

Day 6

1. Blood Cleanser

Juice one whole lemon and add to 200ml (7fl oz) of warm water.

2. Vitamin Vitality Meal

500g (1lb 2oz) grapes

1 grapefruit

Calories: 450

3. Raw Alkaline Mineral Meal

Activator Green Smoothie (see recipe on day 2, page 179)

Calories: 400 (300 without the avocado)

4. Fat-Loss Sugar Meal

Banana Green Smoothie (see recipe on Day 1, page 176)

Calories: 500

5. Hearty Cooked-Fibre Meal

Butternut Squash and Sweet Potato Soup

This is my favourite winter soup and a great hit with my clients, friends and family. If squashes are not in season, simply replace the butternut squash with 5 chopped carrots and an extra sweet potato.

1 large butternut squash, peeled and chopped

2 large sweet potatoes, peeled and chopped

1 onion, finely chopped

400g (14oz) can of chopped tomatoes

1 tbsp wholegrain mustard

1 tsp cumin powder

1 tsp cinnamon powder

2 vegetable stock cubes, crumbled

Dash of balsamic vinegar

Pinch of black pepper

Place the butternut squash, sweet potatoes, onion, tomatoes, mustard, cumin, cinnamon and vegetable stock cubes in a large saucepan. Cover with boiling water, stir well then leave to simmer for about 30 minutes, or until the potatoes and squash are soft. Season with black pepper to taste and serve immediately.

Calories: 700

❧ Alkaline-delicious tip ❧

Most of today's meals are liquid-based, which means they will be easy to digest. It's good to have a day like this every now and again because it gives your digestive system a bit of a break and a chance to remove any toxicity or repair any damage.

❧❧

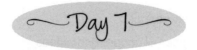

1. Blood Cleanser

Juice one whole lemon and add to 200ml (7fl oz) of warm water.

2. Vitamin Vitality Meal

  2 apples

  2 pears

Calories: 300

3. Raw Alkaline Mineral Meal

Raw Vegetable Crudités and Salsa

Pick five vegetables from the following list and team them with this spicy salsa for a quick, crunchy and colourful snack that will leave you energized. If you're on the go, or if you prefer, you can eat the vegetable crudités for a tasty snack.

  3 florets of broccoli

  3 florets of cauliflower

  2 carrots, sliced into batons

  5 cherry tomatoes

  1 stick celery, sliced into batons

  5cm (2in) stick of cucumber, sliced into batons

  ⅓ red, green or yellow pepper (bell pepper), deseeded and sliced

For the salsa

   1 medium onion, roughly chopped

   3 large tomatoes, roughly chopped

   1 Medjool date, pitted

   Juice of 1 lime

   Handful of fresh coriander (cilantro) leaves

   ½ tsp cayenne pepper

   ½ tsp cumin powder

   Pinch of salt and pepper

Place the onion, tomatoes, date, lime juice, coriander (cilantro) leaves, cayenne pepper and cumin in a blender and blend for 30 seconds, or to your preferred consistency. Season with sea salt to taste. Makes two servings.

Calories: 100 (150 with salsa)

4. Fat-Loss Sugar Meal

   200g (7oz) dates

   5 ripe bananas

Calories: 900

5. Hearty Cooked-Fibre Meal

Baked Potato Wedges

Potatoes are simple, filling and tasty. These are a lovely alternative to chips (fries) and have a lovely crispy texture. Serve with organic tomato ketchup, mustard, chutney (relish) or sweet chilli sauce.

   800g (1lb 12oz) potatoes (uncooked weight), scrubbed and cut into wedges

Preheat the oven to 200°C (400°F or gas mark 6). Place the potatoes in a pan and cover with cold water, bring to the boil then simmer for about 15 minutes or until the potatoes are firm but not soft (parboiled). Drain the potatoes, place on a non-stick baking tray and bake in the oven for 10–15 minutes, turning halfway through cooking for an even brownness. Serve with the condiment of your choice.

Calories: 700

✿ Alkaline-delicious tip ✿

Be kind to yourself and, if possible, take this week easy on the socializing front, so that you can focus your energies on getting to grips with A5D.

✿✿

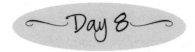

1. Blood Cleanser

Wheatgrass juice (made with 1 tsp of powder in 500ml (18fl oz) of water) or freshly juiced shot

2. Vitamin Vitality Meal

500g (1lb 2oz) grapes

1 grapefruit

Calories: 450

3. Raw Alkaline Mineral Meal

Ginger Activator Green Smoothie (see recipe on Day 2, page 179)

Calories: 400 (300 without the avocado)

4. Fat-Loss Sugar Meal

200g (7oz) dates

Calories: 600

5. Hearty Cooked-Fibre Meal

Alkaline Vegan Porridge

You can make a delicious and warming porridge with oats and either coconut milk or almond milk. Top it with a drizzle of agave syrup or coconut palm sugar for added sweetness.

150g (5½oz) large oats (uncooked weight)

200ml (7fl oz) coconut or almond milk

1 tbsp agave syrup or coconut palm sugar

Pinch of cinnamon powder

Place the oats, coconut milk, agave syrup and cinnamon powder in a saucepan. Bring to the boil, stirring continuously to prevent sticking, then reduce the heat and simmer, and stir for a further 3 minutes or until the porridge is cooked and has a thick, creamy consistency. Place in a bowl and drizzle with a little extra agave syrup or coconut palm sugar, coconut or almond milk, if desired. Enjoy immediately.

Calories: 700

❧ Alkaline-delicious tip ☙

This week, you'll be having wheatgrass juice as your Blood Cleanser, instead of lemon and warm water. So you'll be having an extra daily dose of chlorophyll, which has anti-ageing properties amongst many other benefits and is packed full of minerals.

❧❧

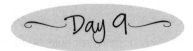

1. Blood Cleanser

Wheatgrass juice (made with 1 tsp of powder in 500ml (18fl oz) of water) or freshly juiced shot

2. Vitamin Vitality Meal

1 litre (1¾ pints) of freshly squeezed orange juice. If you want to make this yourself, rather than buying it, you'll need around 15 oranges.

Calories: 500

3. Raw Alkaline Mineral Meal

Raw Vegetable Crudités and Salsa (see recipe on Day 7, page 192)

Calories: 100 (150 with salsa)

4. Fat-Loss Sugar Meal

5 ripe bananas

Calories: 500

5. Hearty Cooked-Fibre Meal

Vegetable Cumin Buckwheat

Buckwheat is gluten-free, tasty and nutty, and it cooks quickly. It is inexpensive and you can find it in your local health food store or online.

150g (5½oz) buckwheat (uncooked weight)

2 big sprigs of curly or dinosaur kale, finely chopped

3 mushrooms, finely chopped

½ medium onion, finely chopped

3 broccoli florets, finely chopped

2 medium tomatoes, finely chopped

For the sauce

1 vegetable stock cube, crumbled

½ tsp turmeric powder

½ tsp cumin powder

½ tsp cinnamon powder

½ tsp black pepper

1 tbsp agave syrup

250ml (8½fl oz) boiling water

Place the buckwheat in a pan and cover with boiling water then cook according to the packet instructions. In the last 5 minutes of cooking, add the curly kale, mushrooms, onion, broccoli and tomatoes. To make the sauce, add the vegetable stock cube, turmeric, cumin, cinnamon, black pepper and agave syrup to a bowl before pouring in the hot water and stirring well until the stock cube has dissolved. Drain the buckwheat and vegetables, return to the heat and pour over the sauce. Gently mix the sauce into the buckwheat and vegetable mixture, while simmering for a further minute. Serve immediately.

Calories: 700

🌿 Alkaline-delicious tip 🌿

If you had any detox symptoms last week then these should be easing off now and you may be noticing that your clothes feel a little looser.

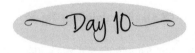

Day 10

1. Blood Cleanser

Wheatgrass juice (made with 1 tsp of powder in 500ml (18fl oz) of water) or freshly juiced shot

2. Vitamin Vitality Meal

1 mango

1 apple

1 pear

200g (7oz) blueberries

Calories: 500

3. Raw Alkaline Mineral Meal

Avocado and Spinach Salad with Asian Dressing

Salads are so versatile and the addition of avocado and this delicious spicy dressing make this salad a warming treat, even on a cold day.

3 large handfuls of spinach leaves

2 medium tomatoes, diced

5cm (2in) cucumber, diced

1 stick celery, finely diced

⅓ red pepper (bell), deseeded and finely sliced

½ avocado, pitted and finely sliced

For the dressing

2 dates, pitted

½ red pepper (bell pepper), deseeded

½ clove of garlic

1¼cm (½in) piece of fresh root ginger

3 tbsp water

Pinch of black pepper

Place the spinach, tomato, cucumber, celery and red pepper (bell pepper) in a large mixing bowl and toss gently to combine. Make the dressing by placing the dates, red pepper (bell pepper), garlic, ginger and water into a blender and blitzing for 1 minute. Season with black pepper to taste. Add the avocado to the salad vegetables then drizzle with dressing. Serve immediately.

Calories: 300

4. Fat-Loss Sugar Meal

Banana Green Smoothie (see recipe on Day 1, page 176)

Calories: 500

5. Hearty Cooked-Fibre Meal

Vegetable Spaghetti Marinara (see recipe on Day 3, page 182)

Calories: 700

🌿 Alkaline-delicious tip 🌿

We only tend to crave what our body already has in it. In the same way that a non-smoker doesn't crave cigarettes, a vegetarian doesn't crave meat. You'll soon get used to satisfying your sugar cravings with dates and bananas.

🌿🌿

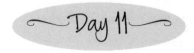

Day 11

1. Blood Cleanser

Wheatgrass juice (made with 1 tsp of powder in 500ml (18fl oz) of water) or freshly juiced shot

2. Vitamin Vitality Meal

500g (1lb 2oz) grapes

1 grapefruit

Calories: 350

3. Raw Alkaline Mineral Meal

Activator Green Smoothie (see recipe on Day 2, page 179)

Calories: 400 (300 without the avocado)

4. Fat-Loss Sugar Meal

Banana 'Nice Cream'

This recipe is a standard vegan secret and means that you don't have to miss out on ice cream if you like it, as this is a really delicious alternative. It tastes surprisingly creamy and just like regular dairy ice cream, but it won't adversely affect your waistline, skin or hormones.

5 ripe bananas, peeled and frozen

50ml (2fl oz) water or coconut water or coconut milk

Dash of natural vanilla extract

1 tsp agave syrup

Place the frozen bananas, water and vanilla extract in a high-speed blender and blitz for 1–2 minutes, or until the consistency is thick and creamy. Serve immediately with agave syrup drizzled over the top

Calories: 600

5. Hearty Cooked-Fibre Meal

Hearty Half-and-Half Mash

400g (14oz) potatoes (uncooked weight), scrubbed and chopped

400g (14oz) sweet potatoes (uncooked weight), scrubbed and chopped

1 vegetable stock cube, crumbled

1 tsp cumin powder

1 tsp cinnamon powder

1 tbsp agave syrup

1 tsp black pepper

Place the potatoes and sweet potatoes in a large saucepan and cover with boiling water. Simmer for 25 minutes or until the potatoes are soft. Drain the potatoes well and then add the vegetable stock cube, cumin, cinnamon and agave syrup. Mash well with a fork and season with black pepper to taste. Serve immediately.

Calories: 700

🌿 Alkaline-delicious tip 🌿

The diet can be as expensive or inexpensive as you would like it to be, but cost should not be an excuse. In fact, you may find that your food bills go down, particularly if you're used to eating a lot of meat and fish.

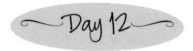

1. Blood Cleanser

Wheatgrass juice (made with 1 tsp of powder in 500ml (18fl oz) of water) or freshly juiced shot

2. Vitamin Vitality Meal

    1 large mango

    2 pears

Calories: 350

3. Raw Alkaline Mineral Meal

Banana Green Smoothie (see recipe on Day 1, page 176)

Calories: 500

4. Fat-Loss Sugar Meal

    100g (3oz) dates

Calories: 300

5. Hearty Cooked-Fibre Meal

Everything Vegetable and Brown (wholegrain) Rice Soup

When root vegetables aren't in season I tend to make an 'everything' vegetable soup, which is really tasty and filling, especially with the addition of some brown (wholegrain) rice. The vegetables in the soup depend on what's in my organic seasonal vegetable box that week, but I usually use a cabbage, a can of chopped tomatoes, an onion and then maybe throw in some aubergine (eggplant), leeks, carrots or courgettes (zucchini). Try this recipe and feel free to add the seasonal vegetables of your choice.

100g (3oz) brown (wholegrain) rice (uncooked weight)

½ small cabbage

2 carrots, scrubbed and chopped

1 leek, sliced

1 onion, chopped

400g (14oz) can of chopped tomatoes

½ aubergine (eggplant), chopped

2 vegetable stock cubes, crumbled

1 tsp wholegrain mustard

1 tsp curry powder

½ tsp black pepper

500ml (18fl oz) boiling water

Place the rice, cabbage, carrots, leek, onion, tomatoes, aubergine (eggplant), stock cubes, wholegrain mustard, curry powder and black pepper in a large saucepan and cover with the boiling water. Stir well then leave to simmer for about 30 minutes. Help yourself to a big bowl or two, and enjoy.

Calories: 700

🌿 Alkaline-delicious tip 🌿

You are over halfway through this 21-day programme. Take a moment to note your achievement so far and do a mental scan of your body for how it's feeling. Have a look in the mirror; can you notice any changes to your weight, skin, hair or eyes?

🌿🌿

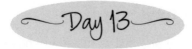

1. Blood Cleanser

Wheatgrass juice (made with 1 tsp of powder in 500ml (18fl oz) of water) or freshly juiced shot

2. Vitamin Vitality Meal

Apple Pomegranate Medley

This is a wonderful breakfast recipe that is zingy and sweet, has great texture, is energizing and is a great alternative to granola, cereal or porridge.

    2 apples, grated
    ½ pomegranate, peeled and deseeded
    Handful of blueberries
    Juice of ½ lemon
    ½ tsp cinnamon powder

Place the apple, pomegranate and blueberries in a large bowl and gently combine with the lemon juice and cinnamon. Place in a bowl and serve immediately.

Calories: 350

3. Raw Alkaline Mineral Meal

You'll eat two smaller 'meals' for your RAMM today.

Mango Tomato Salad

This salad is easy and fast to make and has a clean, sweet taste. Mangoes and tomatoes combine really well together to make a dressing that is full of flavour and will make your salad come alive.

> 2 large handfuls of spinach
>
> 1 large beef tomato or 5 cherry tomatoes, sliced
>
> 5cm (2in) cucumber, finely sliced
>
> ¼ red pepper (bell pepper), deseeded and finely sliced

For the dressing

> ½ mango, peeled, pitted and sliced
>
> 2 medium tomatoes
>
> Pinch of cayenne pepper

Place the spinach, tomato, cucumber and red pepper (bell pepper) in a large mixing bowl and toss gently to combine. To make the dressing, place the mango and tomatoes in a blender and blitz for 1 minute, then season with cayenne pepper to taste. Drizzle the dressing over the salad and gently toss the salad to combine. Serve immediately.

Calories: 300

Ginger Activator Green Smoothie (see recipe on Day 2, page 179)

Calories: 400 (300 without the avocado)

4. Fat-Loss Sugar Meal

> 5 medium bananas

Calories: 500

5. Hearty Cooked-Fibre Meal

Alkaline Vegan Porridge (see recipe on Day 8, page 195)

Calories: 700

Alkaline-delicious tip

If you find you are struggling to explain to other people why you're doing this diet, then you can always say it has been recommended to you by a doctor – and that would be true: doctors Barnard, McDougall, Esselstyn, Campbell and Graham all recommend that everyone should eat this way and you'll find a list of their books in the Resources section on page 231.

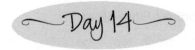

Day 14

1. Blood Cleanser

Wheatgrass juice (made with 1 tsp of powder in 500ml (18fl oz) of water) or freshly juiced shot

2. Vitamin Vitality Meal

2 medium mangoes

Calories: 400

3. Raw Alkaline Mineral Meal

Date Milk Smoothie

If you find it difficult to eat lots of dates or want a drink that really packs in the calories and nutrients, you can't do much better than this smoothie. It's creamy, sweet and makes the perfect sports drink for before, during or after exercise because it's convenient, easily digested and provides instant energy.

10 large Medjool dates, pitted

500ml–1 litre (18fl oz–1¾ pints) water (depending on your preferred consistency)

Place the dates into a blender, cover with 500ml (18fl oz) of the water and blitz for 1 minute. If you prefer a thinner consistency, keep adding liquid (up to 1 litre/1¾ pints) until you reach the consistency you prefer. Pour into a large glass or sports bottle and enjoy.

4. Fat-Loss Sugar Meal

4 medium bananas

Calories: 400

5. Hearty Cooked-Fibre Meal

Mango Millet

Millet is a small, gluten-free grain, similar to quinoa and with a hint of nuttiness and a great texture. For some reason it is one of the least popular grains, but, as you'll discover, millet is a great choice for your daily HCFM and it goes really well with some mango chutney (relish).

150g (5½oz) millet (uncooked weight)

3 mushrooms, diced

5cm (2in) slice of courgette (zucchini), finely diced

For the sauce

2 tbsp mango chutney (relish)

½ tsp cumin powder

Pinch of black pepper

Place the millet in a pan and cover with boiling water then cook for the time specified on the packet instructions. In the last 5 minutes of cooking, add the mushrooms and courgette (zucchini) to the pan. To make the sauce, place the mango chutney (relish) and cumin in a blender and blitz for 30 seconds then season with black pepper to taste. Drain the millet and vegetables, return to the heat and stir in the sauce until well combined. Serve immediately.

Calories: 700

🌿 Alkaline-delicious tip 🌿

Are you remembering to do your other alkaline activities – deep breathing, daily walking and the other things from the Framework for Optimum Health and Healing? Refresh your memory by checking back through Part II of the book again.

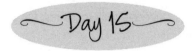

1. Blood Cleanser

Wheatgrass juice (made with 1 tsp of powder in 500ml (18fl oz) of water) or freshly juiced shot

2. Vitamin Vitality Meal

1 litre (1¾ pints) of fresh orange juice. If you want to make this yourself, rather than buying it, you'll need around 15 oranges.

Calories: 500

3. Raw Alkaline Mineral Meal

Raw Vegetable Crudités and Salsa (see recipe on Day 7, page 192)

Calories: 100 (150 with salsa)

4. Fat-Loss Sugar Meal

Persimmon Spice Cake Mix

This recipe is divine! To me it tastes just like the cake mix that my Mum used to make when I was a child that I liked to spoon out of the bowl – but it has none of the fat, dairy or refined sugars. Serve in a bowl as a pudding, or as a smoothie. If persimmons are not in season, use 2 apples instead for an apple-pie flavour.

    1 very ripe persimmon, topped
    6 Medjool dates, pitted
    ½ tsp mixed spice (pumpkin-pie spice)

4 tbsp water or almond milk (optional, for a thinner consistency)

Place the persimmon, dates and mixed spice in a blender and blend for 1 minute. Serve in a pudding bowl. For a thinner consistency (more like a smoothie), add 4 tbsp of water or almond milk and blend for 1 minute. Serve in a tall glass and drink immediately.

5. Hearty Cooked-Fibre Meal

Vegetable Cumin Brown (wholegrain) Rice (see recipe on Day 1, page 176)

Calories: 700

❦ Alkaline-delicious tip ❦

This week, feel free to experiment more with your Hearty Cooked-Fibre Meal; add extra vegetables, try different spices and herbs if you wish. Keep going, I bet you're doing great.

❦❦

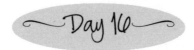

1. Blood Cleanser

Wheatgrass juice (made with 1 tsp of powder in 500ml (18fl oz) of water) or freshly juiced shot

2. Vitamin Vitality Meal

500g (1lb 2oz) grapes

1 grapefruit

Calories: 350

3. Raw Alkaline Mineral Meal

Raw Vegetable Soup

This recipe works well if you have a high-speed blender – you can create a semi-warm vegetable soup by blitzing the vegetables on high for 5 minutes. It is technically raw because it's not heated enough to cook the ingredients and is easier and quicker to prepare than a conventional soup. Simply throw the ingredients into your blender, blend and serve. Try the recipe below, but don't forget to experiment too. To make a raw soup, you just need a leafy green base, two or three other raw veg, some herbs and spices, lemon juice and something to give it a bit more flavour, such as an onion or tomatoes or garlic.

3 large handfuls of leafy greens, such as kale, spinach, chard, watercress, or rocket

½ onion

Juice of ½ lemon

1 medium tomato

1 stalk of celery

100ml (3½fl oz) water

Pinch of cayenne pepper

Pinch of salt and pepper

½ avocado, pitted (optional)

Place all the ingredients in a blender and blitz for 2–3 minutes, or until the soup is your preferred consistency. Add the avocado if you prefer a creamier, richer soup.

Calories: 100 (200 with avocado)

4. Fat-Loss Sugar Meal

Banana Green Smoothie (see recipe on Day 1, page 176)

Calories: 500

5. Hearty Cooked-Fibre Meal

Alkaline Vegan Porridge (see recipe on Day 8, page 195)

Calories: 700

✣ Alkaline-delicious tip ✣

Try cooking a Hearty Cooked-Fibre Meal for your family or friends. You can generally make one of the vegetable and grain meals for less than the price of a loaf of bread per person. Give it a go! If you don't tell them it's alkaline and vegan, it's unlikely they'll even notice that it's a super-healthy way of eating; they'll just say it's tasty.

✣

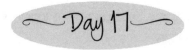

1. Blood Cleanser

Wheatgrass juice (made with 1 tsp of powder in 500ml (18fl oz) of water) or freshly juiced shot

2. Vitamin Vitality Meal

    2 pears

    2 apples

Calories: 300

3. Raw Alkaline Mineral Meal

Raw Vegetable Crudités and Salsa (see recipe on Day 7, page 192)

Calories: 150

4. Fat-Loss Sugar Meal

    200g (7oz) dates

    2 bananas

Calories: 800

5. Hearty Cooked-Fibre Meal

Quinoa with Peas

This adds a nice bit of variety to your HCFM. Peas and quinoa go well together with this simple tomato sauce. Keep quinoa as a staple at home as you're always likely to have the ingredients for this type of recipe and can whip it together quickly when you're feeling hungry.

> 150g (5½ oz) quinoa (uncooked weight)
>
> 100g (3oz) frozen peas
>
> 1 carrot, scrubbed and chopped
>
> 2 medium tomatoes, chopped

For the sauce

> 3 tbsp tomato purée
>
> 1 tbsp agave syrup
>
> ½ tsp dried oregano
>
> ½ tsp dried basil
>
> ½ tsp black pepper

Place the quinoa in a saucepan, cover with boiling water and then cook according to the packet instructions. In the last 5 minutes of cooking add the peas, carrot and tomatoes. To make the sauce place the tomato purée, agave syrup, oregano, basil and black pepper in a bowl and mix well. Drain the quinoa and vegetables well, return to the heat then pour over the sauce and mix for at least 1 minute or until well combined. Serve immediately.

Calories: 700

❧ Alkaline-delicious tip ❧

Keep going until the end of the 21 days, you're doing great. If after the 21 days you carry on with one or two of the meals every day, this would still make a very positive impact on your health.

❧❧

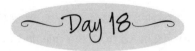

1. Blood Cleanser

Wheatgrass juice (made with 1 tsp of powder in 500ml (18fl oz) of water) or freshly juiced shot

2. Vitamin Vitality Meal

Apple Pomegranate Medley (see recipe on Day 13, page 207)

Calories: 350

3. Raw Alkaline Mineral Meal

Ginger Activator Green Smoothie (see recipe on Day 1, page 179)

Calories: 400 (300 without the avocado)

4. Fat-Loss Sugar Meal

Baked Bananas and 'Caramel' Sauce

These are like the banana fritters that you get in Asian restaurants, but without the saturated or hydrogenated fat and batter. Warm, sweet and gooey. Yum!

    5 ripe bananas, peeled

    3 dates

    2 tbsp water

First make the sauce by placing 1 banana, the dates and the water in a blender and blitzing for 30 seconds. Halve the remaining bananas by cutting them lengthwise, and place under a hot grill (broiler) for 3–4 minutes or until they start to sizzle and brown. Remove from the grill and then drizzle the sauce over the top. Serve immediately.

Calories: 500

5. Hearty Cooked-Fibre Meal

Bulgur Wheat Cabbage Wraps (see recipe on Day 2, page 180)

Calories: 700

🌿 Alkaline-delicious tip 🌿

The low-fat and nutrient-dense meals will be helping you to feel energized. Hopefully you'll notice that you aren't experiencing the afternoon tiredness that so many people experience after lunch.

🌿🌿

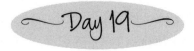

1. Blood Cleanser

Wheatgrass juice (made with 1 tsp of powder in 500ml (18fl oz of water) or freshly juiced shot

2. Vitamin Vitality Meal

2 pears

2 apples

Calories: 300

3. Raw Alkaline Mineral Meal

Banana Mustard Salad

The salad is full of colour and flavour and the banana dressing gives it spicy sweetness.

2 large handfuls of salad leaves

5cm (2in) cucumber, finely sliced

5 baby tomatoes, halved

1 stick celery, finely sliced

1 medium carrot, grated

For the dressing

1 banana, peeled

1 tbsp apple cider vinegar or balsamic vinegar

1 tbsp agave syrup

1 tbsp wholegrain mustard

1 tsp cumin powder

300ml (10fl oz) water

Pinch of black pepper

Place the salad leaves, cucumber, tomato, celery and carrot in a large mixing bowl and gently toss to combine. To make the dressing, place the banana, apple cider vinegar, agave syrup, cumin and water into a blender and blitz for 2 minutes. Season with pepper to taste. Drizzle the dressing over the salad and gently toss to combine. Serve immediately.

Calories: 300

4. Fat-Loss Sugar Meal

200g (7oz) dates

Calories: 600

5. Hearty Cooked-Fibre Meal

Hearty Half-and-Half Mash (see recipe on Day 11 page 203)

Calories: 700

✵ Alkaline-delicious tip ✵

When you're out and about or food shopping, keep a lookout for food brands that may be compatible with A5D and then you can include them in your everyday food choices after these 21 days, if you want. Dried fruits, rice cakes and corn crackers can all make tasty snacks.

✵✵✵

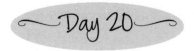

1. Blood Cleanser

Wheatgrass juice (made with 1 tsp of powder in 500ml (18fl oz) of water) or freshly juiced shot

2. Vitamin Vitality Meal

Apple Pomegranate Medley (see recipe on Day 13, page 207)

Calories: 350

3. Raw Alkaline Mineral Meal

Ginger Activator Green Smoothie (see recipe on Day 2, page 179)

Calories: 400 (300 without the avocado)

4. Fat-Loss Sugar Meal

Banana 'Nice Cream' (see recipe on Day 11, page 202)

Calories: 600

5. Hearty Cooked-Fibre Meal

Sweet Chilli Asian Noodles

This lovely noodle dish uses tamari soy sauce for the first time. Tamari is similar to soy sauce and it's much easier to find an organic version than soy sauce, which is important since most non-organic soy is GMO. You'll be able to cook this in a matter of minutes and it tastes authentically Asian.

150g (5½ oz) wholegrain noodles or spaghetti (uncooked weight)

½ onion, peeled and finely chopped

½ red pepper (bell pepper), deseeded and finely chopped

3 florets of broccoli, chopped

3 mushrooms, sliced

For the sauce

1 tbsp sweet chilli sauce

1 tbsp tamari

1 tbsp agave syrup

1cm (½ in) piece of fresh root ginger, peeled and finely sliced, or pinch of ground ginger powder

Pinch of black pepper

Place the noodles, onion, red pepper (bell pepper), broccoli and mushrooms in a large saucepan and cover with boiling water, then cook according to the noodle packet instructions. To make the sauce, place the chilli sauce, tamari, agave syrup, ginger and black pepper in a bowl and combine well. Drain the noodles and vegetables, return to the heat, then add the sauce and gently mix together well for about a minute. Serve immediately.

Calories: 700

✺ Alkaline-delicious tip ✺

Eat more: remember, you need to think *volume* on this diet, which you will quickly get used to – it's just a simple mindset shift.

✵✵✵

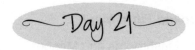

1. Blood Cleanser

Wheatgrass juice (made with 1 tsp of powder in 500ml (18fl oz) of water) or freshly juiced shot

2. Vitamin Vitality Meal

500g (1lb 2oz) grapes

1 grapefruit

Calories: 450

3. Raw Alkaline Mineral Meal

Ginger Activator Green Smoothie (see page 179)

Calories: 400 (300 without the avocado)

4. Fat-Loss Sugar Meal

Banana Smoothie

This is a standard banana smoothie – sweet, delicious and very satisfying. Some people find fully ripe bananas a bit too sweet, but blended they taste like a banana milkshake.

5 medium bananas

100ml (3½fl oz) coconut water or coconut milk

2 large or 4 small dates, pitted (optional)

Place the ingredients into a blender and blitz for about 30 seconds. Pour into a glass and drink immediately.

Calories: 550 (650 with the dates)

5. *Hearty Cooked-Fibre Meal*

Couscous with Mushrooms and Mango

When you are really hungry or don't have time to cook, this recipe is your quick and easy solution. It's very tasty too, with gorgeous Moroccan flavours.

150g (5½oz) couscous (uncooked weight)

3 mushrooms, finely chopped

¼ onion, finely chopped

20g (1oz) raisins

½ tsp cumin powder

1 vegetable stock cube dissolved in 175ml (6fl oz) boiling water

Pinch of black pepper

1 tbsp mango chutney

Place the couscous, mushrooms, onion, raisins and cumin into a saucepan and cover with the vegetable stock. Simmer for 5 minutes, stirring continuously, until the water is dissolved. Turn off the heat, cover and leave for 5 minutes to steam, then fork through the grains to loosen and fluff them. Season with black pepper and serve with a dollop of mango chutney (relish).

Calories: 700

❧ Alkaline-delicious tip ❧

You did it. Well done! How do you feel? Write down what you loved about the past 21 days. Go to our online community detailed on page 231 in the Resources section and let us know about your experience and your results.

❧❧

Conclusion

Moving Forward: Staying Alkaline

Now that you've completed 21 days on A5D, I encourage you to continue with it. This diet is very much sustainable over the long term. Remember, I created and refined it to meet five specific criteria:

1. Simple

2. Satisfying

3. Super-healthy

4. Sustainable

5. Systematized

As long as you eat one of each of the five meals each day, there is a lot of flexibility. Experiment all you want with fruit and green smoothies and with your Hearty Cooked-Fibre Meals by adding different vegetables and grains and spices.

❧ Alkaline-delicious tip ❧

Remember, it's important to eat enough. Monitor your calories to make sure you're not under-eating, which is all too easy on a plant-based diet.

Final thoughts

You may have noticed throughout your life things that simply haven't worked out that well when it comes to your diet and lifestyle; maybe even your overall health and physical condition. Many of these things will be due to the long-held habits that you've engaged in. It could be those few glasses of red wine after work on Friday evenings, or that lunchtime chocolate bar, or the ice cream while watching TV, or daily meat-based meals.

The Alkaline 5 Diet offers you a refreshingly different and healthier way of living and eating and, if you've now completed the 21-day programme, I'm sure you've already experienced some great benefits.

The tendency however, may be to go back to some old habits that do not serve you or your health. I want you to be mindful of these and I urge you to keep up many of the new habits and meals that you've discovered.

Don't let old mindsets and bad foods creep back in. Don't let other people's views put you off. Don't waste your time and health with other diets. The majority of people you and I know are unhealthy and will be battling with some kind of preventable disease in their lifetime, if not already, so don't let their misplaced views sway you.

If you need to add leverage to committing to this lifestyle then you may want to check out some animal rights documentaries, like *Earthlings*, to bring the ethical angle into the mix too.

Embrace this lifestyle and you will reap a multitude of benefits over the long term, as well as the short term, just like sustained exercise over a period of years *really* sculpts your body and fitness, as well as giving you a great initial kick if you do it for a few weeks.

We are living in seriously unhealthy times and environments. The Alkaline 5 Diet and the seven principles of the Framework to Optimum Health and Healing offer you a lifeline and an insurance policy for achieving and keeping great health, a great body and a great mind. Take action now to secure the health of you and your family; don't get entangled in the downward spiral of the medical system.

Have a look back over the framework (see page 53) and write down two new goals, action or habits for each of seven areas. Commit to sticking to these for 30 days and then, at the end of that period, review them and update them for the next 30 days. This will really help to keep you focused on the path of great health.

Sharing A5D

As we've come to the end of this book and our time together here, I'd like to tell you how grateful I am to be able to share this diet and ideas with you and I sincerely hope that you can experience a level of health and happiness that surpasses what you've been used to.

The information in this book has created magnificence in my own life and in the lives of other people who have so kindly emailed to let me know how it's worked for them. I know it can work for you, too, and you can experience the pure joy of being lean, fit and healthy.

Please do let your friends, family and colleagues know about this book and engage with my online community and other people who are following A5D; I'd love to hear from you and continue to provide you with resources to help you.

Remember to get your free, full-colour A5D printable wall chart and video guide from me at www.Alkaline5Diet.com. Use the password laurawilson.

Wishing you great health, a fit body, a positive and happy mind and an abundance of fruits and vegetables.

God bless,

Laura Wilson

Resources

Since you bought this book, you are entitled to get a free copy of my full-colour Alkaline 5 Diet handy info-graphic that you can print and put on your wall or have on your desktop as an easy referral guide to help you succeed with A5D. You also get a free video guide that I've recorded for you. Simply go to:

www.Alkaline5Diet.com and use the password: laurawilson

My site also features articles and information about one-to-one coaching and where to buy equipment, foods and supplements.

Documentaries

Breaking the Food Seduction (2011), Dr Neal Barnard (Based on his 2003 book of the same name)

Earthlings (2005)

Fighting the Big Fat Lies with The Fad Free Truth (2004), Dr John McDougall (series of 11 interesting lectures)

Food Matters (2008)

Forks Over Knives (2011)

Books

Foods That Fight Pain (1998), Dr Neal Barnard

Turn Off the Fat Genes (2001), Dr Neal Barnard

Program for Reversing Diabetes (2007), Dr Neal Barnard

The China Study (2005), Dr T Colin Campbell

The Starch Solution (2012), Dr John McDougall

Prevent and Reverse Heart Disease (2008), Dr Caldwell Esselstyn

Eat More, Weigh Less (2001), Dr Dean Ornish

The 80/10/10 Diet (2006), Dr Doug Graham

Be Your Own Doctor (1975), Ann Wigmore

Wheatgrass: Nature's Finest Medicine (2007), Steve Meyerowitz

Websites

www.Alkaline5Diet.com – book and health website

www.laurawilsononline.com – my personal website

www.nealbarnard.org – Dr Neal Barnard

www.juicemaster.com – Jason Vale

Endnotes

Introduction: Welcome to Abundance, Balance and Harmony

1. http://www.who.int/mediacentre/factsheets/fs311/en/ [accessed 12 October 2014]

Chapter 1: The Good and Bad News about Diet and Health

1. http://www.corporatewatch.org.uk/content/corporate-watch-food-drink-federation-influence-lobbying#gov [accessed 12 Oct 2014]
2. http://www.ion.ac.uk/information/onarchives/vitamincontroversy [accessed 12 October 2014]
3. http://www.hsph.harvard.edu/nutritionsource/calcium-full-story/ [accessed 12 October 2014]
4. Barnard, N. *Turn off the Fat Genes* (Harmony/Random House, 2001)
5. http://rt.com/usa/gmo-gluten-sensitivity-trigger-343/ [accessed 10 October 2014]
6. http://responsibletechnology.org/media/images/content/Press_Release_Gluten_11_25.pdf [accessed 10 November 2014]
7. http://www.sciencedirect.com/science/article/pii/S0278691512005637 [accessed 10 November 2014]
8. http://www.ncbi.nlm.nih.gov/pubmed/23756170 [accessed 10 November 2014]
9. http://earthopensource.org/files/pdfs/Roundup-and-birth-defects/RoundupandBirthDefectsv5.pdf [accessed 10 November 2014]
10. Warburg, O. 'The Prime Cause and Prevention of Cancer', Lecture delivered to Nobel Laureates at Lindau, Lake Constance, Germany, 30 June, 1966
11. http://mosao2.org/Article%20-%20Medicine/cancer_Otto_Warburg_00.pdf [accessed 12 November 2014]
12. http://en.wikipedia.org/wiki/S._P._L._S%C3%B8rensen [accessed 10 November 2014]
13. http://www.ion.ac.uk/information/onarchives/alkaline [accessed 10 November 2014]
14. Lanou, A. and Castleman, A. *Building Bone Vitality* (McGraw-Hill Contemporary; 1st edition, 2009)

15. http://www.biotherapy-clinic.com/alkalize.html [accessed 10 November 2014]
16. http://hippocratesinst.org/the-institute/ann-wigmore-founder [accessed 12 October 2014]
17. Young, R. *The pH Miracle Balance* (Piatkus, 2009)
18. Vasey, C. *The Acid–Alkaline Diet for Optimum Heath* (Healing Arts Press; 2nd Revised edition, 2006)
19. Padden Jubb, A. *Secrets of an Alkaline Body* (North Atlantic Books; Reprint edition, 2004)
20. http://news.harvard.edu/gazette/2003/03.13/09-kidney.html [accessed 12 October 2014]
21. http://www.medicalnewstoday.com/articles/271663.php [accessed 12 October 2014]
22. https://www.drmcdougall.com/misc/2007nl/apr/protein.htm [accessed 12 October 2014]

(Part I) Introduction: Essential Elements for Health

1. Tomljenovic, L. 'Aluminum and Alzheimer's Disease: After a Century of Controversy, Is there a Plausible Link?' *Alzheimer's Disease,* 2010; 23: 567–98
2. Barr, L. Metaxas, G. *et al.* 'Measurement of Paraben Concentrations in Human Breast Tissue at Serial Locations Across the Breast from Axilla to Sternum', *Journal of Applied Toxicology,* 2012; 32(3): 219–32

Chapter 4: A Big Breath of Fresh Air: Deep Oxygenation

1. http://en.wikipedia.org/wiki/Cellular_respiration [accessed 12 October 2014]
2. http://en.wikipedia.org/wiki/Warburg_hypothesis [accessed 12 October 2014]

Chapter 5: Plump your Cells, Lubricate your Brain

1. http://www.medicaldaily.com/75-americans-may-suffer-chronic-dehydration-according-doctors-247393 [accessed 12 October 2014]
2. http://www.alive.com/articles/view/17570/are_you_chronically_dehydrated [accessed 12 October 2014]
3. http://www.nlm.nih.gov/medlineplus/ency/article/002471.htm [accessed 12 October 2014]
4. http://www.brainfacts.org/brain-basics/neural-network-function/articles/2008/the-neural-regulation-of-thirst// [accessed 12 October 2014]
5. http://drsircus.com/medicine/water/dehydration-3 [accessed 12 October 2014]
6. http://water.epa.gov/drink/contaminants/ [accessed 12 October 2014]

7. http://www.nrdc.org/water/drinking/uscities.asp [accessed 12 October 2014]
8. http://water.epa.gov/drink/contaminants/ [accessed 12 October 2014]
9. http://www.nrdc.org/water/drinking/uscities.asp [accessed 12 October 2014]
10. http://articles.mercola.com/sites/articles/archive/2013/12/24/fluoride-toxicity.aspx [accessed 12 October 2014]
11. Kouchakoff, P. 'The Influence of Food on the Blood Formula of Man', First International Congress of Microbiology, Paris, 1930

Chapter 6: Dreams Abounding: Sleep and Balancing Rest

1. http://articles.mercola.com/sites/articles/archive/2012/04/09/dr-rubin-naiman-on-how-much-sleep-do-you-need.aspx [accessed 12 October 2014]
2. Hung, C., Anderson, C., Horne, J., McEvoy, P. 'Mobile phone "talk-mode" signal delays EEG-determined sleep onset', *Neurosci Lett.* 21 Jun 2007; 421(1): 82–6. Epub 2007 May 24
3. http://www.memoryfoammattress-guide.org/off-gassing-and-memory-foam/ [accessed 12 October 2014]
4. http://www.myessentia.com/learn/the-icky-truth/list-of-chemicals-in-mattresses/ [accessed 12 October 2014]

Chapter 7: Live and Let Live: Living Alkaline Foods

1. http://www.biotherapy-clinic.com/alkalize.html [accessed 12 October 2014]
2. Lindlahr, V. *You Are What You Eat* (National Nutrition Society, Inc, 1942)
3. http://foodnsport.com/index.php [accessed 12 October 2014]
4. http://hippocratesinst.org/living-food/benefits-of-wheatgrass [accessed 12 October 2014]
5. http://nutritionstudies.org/animal-vs-plant-protein/ [accessed 12 October 2014]
6. http://hippocratesinst.org/the-institute/ann-wigmore-founder [accessed 12 October 2014]

Chapter 8: Ditch the Nasties: Eliminating Acidic Toxins

1. http://caloriecount.about.com/forums/motivation/water-vs-coke-off [accessed 12 October 2014]
2. http://phmiracleliving.com/t-faq-fat.aspx [accessed 12 October 2014]
3. http://nutritionfacts.org/2011/09/08/how-much-pus-is-there-in-milk [accessed 10 November 2014]
4. http://www.channing.harvard.edu [accessed 10 November 2014]

5. http://articles.mercola.com/sites/articles/archive/2014/03/22/
    aluminum-toxicity-alzheimers.aspx [accessed 10 November 2014]
6. http://articles.mercola.com/sites/articles/archive/2010/07/13/sodium-
    lauryl-sulfate.aspx [accessed 10 November 2014]
7. http://www.health-science.com/microwave_hazards.html [accessed
    12 October 2014]
8. http://www.fluoridation.com/c-country.htm [accessed 12 October
    2014]
9. http://www.globalhealingcenter.com/natural-health/10-shocking-
    facts-health-dangers-wifi/ [accessed 12 October 2014]
10. http://www.ncbi.nlm.nih.gov/pubmed/24138364 [accessed
    12 October 2014]

Chapter 10: The Bright Side of Life: Positive Mindset and Emotions

1. http://www.phmiracleliving.com/t-faq-emotions.aspx [accessed
    12 October 2014]

Chapter 11: The Basics of the Alkaline 5 Diet

1. http://pcrm.org/shop/byNealBarnard/turn-off-the-fat-genes
    [accessed 12 October 2014]
2. http://en.wikipedia.org/wiki/Cellular_respiration [accessed
    12 October 2014]
3. http://care.diabetesjournals.org/content/29/8/1777.abstracthttp
    [accessed 12 October 2014]
4. http//www.nealbarnard.org/books/diabetes/ [accessed 12 October
    2014]

Chapter 12: The Alkaline 5 Diet Meals

1. http://www.bmi-calculator.net/bmr-calculator/harris-benedict-
    equation/ [accessed 12 October 2014]
2. http://www.acsm.org/access-public-information/acsm%27s-sports-
    performance-center/factors-that-influence-daily-calorie-needs
    [accessed 12 October 2014]
3. http://www.hc-sc.gc.ca/fn-an/pubs/securit/2012-allergen_sulphites-
    sulfites/index-eng.php [accessed 12 October 2014]
4. http://www.worldhealth.net/news/potassium/ [accessed 12 October
    2014]
5. http://www.nutrition-and-you.com/dates.html [accessed 12 October
    2014
6. Campbell, T.C., Schurman, J. and Campbell, T. *The China Study*
    (BenBella Books; 1st edition, 2006)
7. http://www.naturalnews.com/035632_music_sound_healing_
    medicine.html [accessed 10 November 2014]

ABOUT THE AUTHOR

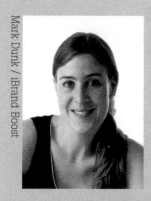

Mark Dunk / iBrand Boost

Laura Wilson is an experienced health coach and competitive athlete. She is a trained nutritionist who has been researching nutrition and natural health since 1999, and truly knows the simple secrets to achieving optimum physical wellbeing, no matter what the starting point.

As a university student, Laura transformed her own health from an overweight, unfit smoker to a lean, vibrant, ultra-marathon runner. She has since helped thousands of people around the world to naturally improve their health, get in great shape, look younger and, in some cases, heal disease.

Laura is a former Medical Research Manager for the National Health Service, a qualified advanced gym and dance instructor and the organizer of the Natural Health and Vitality Conference. Her years of experience in different fields of health and coaching have given Laura a unique and deep insight into what it takes to truly thrive in the unhealthy world we live in.

www.laurawilsononline.com